MUD AND THE CITY

MUD AND THE CITY

Jessica Fellowes

Book Guild Publishing
Sussex, England

First published in Great Britain in 2008 by
The Book Guild Ltd
Pavilion View
19 New Road
Brighton, BN1 1UF

Typesetting in Garamond by
Keyboard Services, Luton, Bedfordshire

Printed in Great Britain by
CPI Antony Rowe

A catalogue record for this book is available from
The British Library

ISBN 978 1 84624 278 6

For
Georgie
Rory
Cordelia
&
Simon

Contents

Summer

CONTENTS

Autumn

Winter

CONTENTS

Acknowledgements

This book wouldn't have happened without several wonderful people, to all of whom I have vast oceans of gratitude for their belief in me. Without their pushing, this book would still be a mere idea. So first to Damian Barr – adorio. To Bridget Harrison and Stefano Hatfield of *The London Paper* for having the wit to see it could be a column first. To Carol Biss of Book Guild, as well as Laura Lockington, Joanna Bentley and Max Crisfield, who all turned it into a real live book.

Thank you to all at *Country Life* for putting up with ridiculous questions ('but what *is* the difference between straw and hay?'), especially Mark Hedges, Clive Aslet, Rupert Uloth, Jane Watkins, Kate Green and Arabella Youens. Thank you, too, to several people who helped answer everything else: Julian Seaman, Marc Randle, Sue Tolson, Jack Wall, Lucy Reeves, Claire Driver, David Profumo, Tessa Waugh and Dylan Williams. Any wrong answers you find here are my fault entirely.

To Clare Penate, the best friend. To Julian and Emma Kitchener-Fellowes, who began teaching me the dos and don'ts from dot. To my sister, Cordelia, for laughing out loud. To my darling mother, Georgie. To my father, Rory, who not only did all a parent should (and more) but was invaluable in making this book as sharp as it can be. To Simon, without whom none of it happens. Thank you.

Introduction

You might consider yourself a hardened townie with brick dust in your veins, and a stronger dependency on carbon monoxide than oxygen for survival. Your hands were made for hailing taxis, not for digging up spuds. Yet vast numbers of townies share one common fantasy: to escape to the country. Some will only want to go for a day, in search of the perfect pub. Some will go for a country wedding or at the behest of their friends who have 'green-shifted' and made the leap from a minimalist chic flat in town to a muddied, messy, roses-around-the-door cottage. The fit ones, or the corporate players, may want to take up shooting or hunting (the old boy network is strong in these quarters). Others still just want a new place to go shopping.

But townies and their country cousins are a divided family under one nation. Townies think country people are either village idiots or land-grabbing toffs. Meanwhile, rural dwellers think townies are ill-informed meddlers passing laws that infringe on the rustic way of life. Either that or they're buying overpriced cottages they only stay in at the weekend.

Now, for the first time, it looks like things are changing. Most significantly, the twenty-first century has brought to the forefront the issues of global warming and climate change: we are having to rethink the food we eat, where we holiday and how we produce fuel. If you are someone who makes the effort to buy organic or local food, you will most likely know the name of the farm your chicken was raised on and have grown to love the misshapen fruit and veg of the farmers' markets. Townies are waking up to the idea that it's only by living off the land that we can save it.

Whilst townies have begun to embrace British produce, there has been a litany of countryside scares – foot-and-mouth disease, bird flu, flooding – which have made many wary of venturing out to explore our green and pleasant fields. But the relentless pressure urbanites live under has not abated, and the dream of seeing one's days out quietly in a secluded spot somewhere remains undimmed. In the last ten years or so, more than two million people have left London for other parts of Britain and one set of statistics predicts the market for second homes will grow by 24% in the next decade. The population is green-shifting, moving out of the mean streets and into the muddy paths. If this is to be a success, the cousins need to try to understand each other. I hope this book helps.

Can you answer these questions?

(Answers at the back. No peeking.)

1. **A farmers' market is:**

   a) A market for farmers to find a wife
   b) A market for townies to buy food from farmers
   c) A market held on a farm

2. **'Badminton' is:**

   a) A tennis-like game with flimsy rackets and a shuttlecock
   b) A stately home that hosts horse trials alongside a shopping extravaganza
   c) A country in Eastern Europe that supplies most of the countryside's domestic staff

3. **If you go through a door marked 'Private' in a National Trust house, you might:**

   a) Startle the family who are quietly having tea in their own home
   b) Set off an alarm that sounds like a ship's horn
   c) Walk into the National Trust offices

4. **At a country house car boot sale, you are likely to find:**

   a) The stately home's cleaner selling illegal cigarettes out of the back of her Ford Fiesta

b) Stella McCartney and Gwyneth Paltrow's cast-offs/presents they gave Mrs Ritchie

c) Lady Toff of Toffington's childhood rocking horse and chucked chintz

5. **When driving, the acceptable country way to say hello to a passing car or walker is:**

   a) Wind down the window, toot the horn and yell 'Ahoy there!'

   b) Slowly raise four fingers off the steering wheel and nod your head very slightly

   c) Wave just like the Queen

6. **You know a country antique shop is the real thing because:**

   a) A bell tinkles above the door when you walk in

   b) When you ask the price, the owner says, 'Ah, well, I saw you coming...'

   c) They sell toby jugs and nothing else

7. **A real music festival in the country is:**

   a) Glastonbury – mud, hippies, electro-pop, tents and pills

   b) Highclere Castle – picnic tables, chairs, chinos, Bryan Ferry and aspirin

   c) When the dogs howl in the middle of the night

8. **A good present to take a host is:**

   a) A hand-tied bouquet

b) Nothing at all
c) A big box of hand-made chocolates

So ... how did you do?

Not to worry.
This book will give you all the answers.

And a thousand others besides.

SPRING

1

Bareback Adventures

Riding

When I was a small child, my father insisted that I learn how to ride. In case, he said, there was an apocalypse and the only means of transport was to jump on the back of a horse and gallop to safety. This despite the fact that we lived in Deptford, a dank corner of south-east London. It would have made more sense to learn to swim the Thames.

I never fully mastered the art of controlling the four-legged beast and finally fell off for the last time, years later, into a ditch in Sussex, my horse having decided it was far safer to follow the speeding mare ahead (which my rosette-covered friend rode) than to obey any of my administrations. But there is still a part of me that yearns for a romantic ride across open fields, in sexy jodhpurs and riding boots. And I can think of nothing better than doing so in the spring, as the country begins its rebirthing process; riding is just the right speed between walking and the car, and you can see up close the fluctuations of the land.

Riding – never 'horseback riding' as advertised in hotel brochures – is still the principal sport of countrymen and women. Sitting at my desk before a window in Suffolk, I see horses and their riders trot by several times a day.

As with most things in life, you can spot who's who by the clothes they wear. Grooms, out exercising their charges (sometimes one or two more in addition to the one they are riding), are easily spotted by their brightly coloured silk caps (called 'silks'), worn over crash hats. They'll also wear a vividly coloured fleece, soft trousers (no jeans, as they chafe horribly) and half-chaps. These riders almost certainly work in a livery stable or a racing yard.

The townies riding their horses past my window give themselves away by their smart velvet riding hats (in black, navy or pale grey), a tweed jacket and jodhpurs. But all riders – town or country, professional or amateur – must wear boots with a heel. Wellies or trainers will slip through the stirrup, and if the wearer falls off, they will almost certainly be dragged.

If you are a weekender in the country but wish to ride your own horse, you can opt for full livery. This is the equivalent of living in a suite at The Ritz: the horses are cared for day and night, and you need only show up for the ride, having paid a huge cheque (about £120 to £150 a week). There is also the option of DIY livery: more B&B than five-star hotel (about £25 to £40 a week). The horses stay in the stables but you do the mucking out, grooming, feeding and exercising.

Whether preparing for an apocalypse, or simply

hankering for a romantic gallop, you must have some lessons first. Basic control of the horse is essential, and if you are going to go on the road (which you will almost inevitably do – few farmers are keen on horses stamping all over their fields, unless they have given permission for a hunt, or it is a permitted bridlepath) you need to know the riders' highway code. Good livery stables, from where you may 'borrow' a horse for a day or two, will assess your riding ability before lending you one of their charges. Watch out, however, if you haven't been on a horse for a while. One friend had an alarming experience when she tried to impress a boyfriend as she performed a rising-trot on a 17.2hh thoroughbred, in front of 8 people, having not been on a horse for 12 years. She also noted that her expensively groomed hair, carefully preened for the date, wilted under the sweaty assault of the borrowed riding hat.

If you are clambering aboard a four-legged beast for the first time, I would recommend that you don't begin with a thoroughbred. It's like a learner driver taking lessons in a Ferrari. Far better to ride a cob, a friendly, sturdy horse that looks after its passengers.

Despite their size and snorts of steam, horses are sensitive creatures. Did you know, for instance, that if they think their rider has died they will not go faster than a trot, for fear of him falling off? Nor will they trample on any bodies lying on the ground beneath them if they can possibly help it (a good fact for protestors to know, when threatened by policemen on horseback). Horses respond to care, stroking of the neck and being talked to. But never stand behind a horse, as they can kick out without realising you are there. If you want to give the nag a little treat, feed him a carrot or Polo mint with your hand flat, or your thumb will disappear in his maw.

If you wish to make friends, a horse will enable you. In any village, you will find a horsey sub-society. It's worth seeking it out, as the members are generally a sociable lot, more often than not they hunt (see chapter 35) and consequently throw a lot of fund-raising parties, which are a sure-fire way to get to know a large number of your new neighbours.

Even children in the country begin their social lives around the local Pony Club. As members, they will not only meet other kids who live close by, but go off on camping weekends, take part in competitions and learn the discipline of caring for a horse and being a part of a team. However, few boys take part: all those young girls together, in love with their horses, make for too many hormones in one room. The real competition, however, doesn't take place in the fields between the riders. It's between the Pony Club mothers, a renowned group of pushy parents, who will urge on their young Ruperts and Hermiones as if training for the Olympics. Don't stand too close to one as she watches her charge go round the jumps – her arms will flail in excitement and her legs can kick out as viciously as a horse's.

Some basic facts you need to know, particularly if you desire to converse with the horse lovers. Horses are measured in hands. One hand is 4 inches, and you measure from the ground to the horse's 'withers' (the bump at the base of its neck). A very big horse is 17hh; a very small horse is 15hh, and ponies are anything below this. (In other words, ponies are not baby horses, a commonly made mistake – baby horses are foals.) A male horse is a horse and a female, a mare. A nag is your wife. You sit on the saddle, hold the reins and the bridle is the network of leather straps over the horse's face. The steel bit goes between the teeth and it is the jerking of this by the reins that largely controls the horse. That, and squeezing its sides with your legs to make it go faster. I point this out because if your horse does a runner, with you on the back, the temptation is to lean forward and grip it between your legs (which will shoot back over its ribcage and tickle it), to try not to fall off. This will only make you go faster than Frankie Dettori (hence me falling off into a ditch). By the way, if someone tells you 'my horse has broken down', this isn't an unsentimental reference to a living beast, but a common phrase, meaning that their horse is no longer fit for riding and must now live out the rest of its days grazing in a field. It is likely that when the motorcar came along, the phrase was simply switched across.

One last point, if you're the one in a car and not on a horse, always, *always* slow down for the riders. Crawl at just 5 mph as you go past and don't speed up until you are a little way ahead. Riders must always say thank you and both parties can enjoy the moment of elegance and good manners that rarely occurs in town.

DO

Borrow a horse before you buy one – teenagers away at boarding school will appreciate their pet being exercised during term time, or a livery stable may lend you a horse for a day.

Wear your own riding hat – the stink of formerly sweaty jockeys is not pleasant on townie-groomed hair.

Wear chaps – leather ones, not gentlemen – for that extra protection of your soft inner thighs.

DON'T

Wear jeans for riding if you don't want to spend the rest of the weekend rubbing Vaseline on your chafed privates.

Lean forward and grip the beast between your legs – unless you are urging the steed to win the Derby.

2

Where Market Forces Rule

Farmers' Markets

Unless you've been living in a plastic (non-recyclable) box for some time, it will be hard to ignore the urgent messages all around telling you to buy organic food, food with no air miles, free-range eggs and beef sliced from a cow that had a life of pure joy and happiness in green fields, and was christened Fred.

But the issues surrounding food labelling ('Made in Britain' can mean little more than that the goods were packaged in the UK, after being grown halfway across the world), and battery eggs masquerading as free-range, has made many people wary of the stuff in shops. If you really care, you need to go back to the farm.

Farmers' markets are dead trendy, I know. But I'm not talking about poncing around in some fancy city centre: the real deal is in the country. Those charming figures leaning on gate posts chewing straw and pointing you in the direction of the field with a bull in it when you get lost – a.k.a. farmers – have had a rough ride. Workers of the land were left desperate and destitute by the nineties passion for importing exotic out-of-season produce (strawberries in January? What were we thinking?), butter mountains, mad cows and the foot-and-mouth crisis in 2001. But if there's one thing the country understands, it's community. Villagers rallied round and began farmers' markets, giving the men who plough and the women who make dough a chance to sell their produce directly to the people. Bypassing often crippling deals with large supermarket chains and avoiding the cruelty of trucking small animals hundreds of miles across country leads to tastier food for your plate.

It's not just the delicious taste of smugness that you feel on your tongue when you buy from these stalls – it's homemade cheese, fluffy bread made from real grain, plump tomatoes and those juicy slices of Fred. Food sold at country farmers' markets should come from within a 50-mile radius and the producers, or members of their family, have to man the stalls. This means that each purchase can take a while: you have to have a little chat about each brown paper bag of goodies. You can ask questions about the happy life of Betty the hen, and the farmer might even show you a picture of her in his wallet.

Each stall sets out a paper plate with samples of food, and if you're a student, or just a Scrooge, you can eat a full three-course meal without paying a penny by going around all the stalls. And have an open mind – at a farmers' market you might find ostrich steaks, soft cheese produced in a Hampshire barn and boar sausages. Make sure you get there in the morning, as there's a limited amount of produce, and it all gets sold quickly. Take plenty of cash and your own shopping bag. Plan your shopping diary carefully, too. Yokels shop at a slower pace and farmers grow their crops even more slowly. Hence farmers' markets tend to follow a convoluted schedule – some may only appear on the second and fourth Saturdays of the month. Other than that, there's not much excuse for not popping along. Go on. Be a happy shopper.

DO

Take your own shopping bags.

Taste the samples on display and get your lunch for free.

Ask the farmers how the produce made it from barn to stall.

Check when the markets are open.

DON'T

Put on an 'amusing' bumpkin accent when talking to the stallholders.

3

Lovejoy

Antique Hunting

Why do we all love the *Antiques Roadshow*? It's not Fiona Bruce's winning smile, or the dodgy bow-ties of the porcelain expert: it's that look of shock on the granny's face when she discovers that the old mug she'd been using as a toothbrush holder is in fact a rare Ming miniature vase and worth enough to take her and a bingo hall of friends on a Saga cruise. We've all had a rummage in the cupboard under the stairs in the hope of finding a similar treasure. Of course, in our tiny townie homes bought for premium prices, spare space is no bigger than a shoebox and unlikely to yield much in the way of Ming. You need to go shopping.

Forget Portobello Road or Brighton's cobbled lanes and their overpriced market stalls with 'olde brasses' for the tourists, or any number of Glaswegian 'design centres' and their reclaimed tat. Get thee to the villages, my friend.

The cheapest finds are in antique flea-markets, which

tend to be held in church halls and are fairly ad-hoc affairs. I love these. On one trestle table you'll find a seasoned seller with enamelled tin jugs, tea towels and, yes, those olde brasses. The next stall along will have what appears to be the last remains of Great Aunt Matilda's legacy – fifties plastic necklaces, fingerless lace gloves and a chipped tea set. You can pick up knick-knacks here, good for making a home look lived in and enough of a bargain to break, or even deliberately smash, during a blazing row or Greek wedding.

But the proper antiques can only be found in proper antique shops. You know they're the real thing because a little bell tinkles when you open the door. Antique hotspots around the country are: Hungerford, West Berkshire; Marlborough, Wiltshire; Harrogate, Yorkshire; and the Cotswolds and Thames Valley areas generally. But be aware that these places have been plundered many times over, and you may be in with more of a chance of coming across a rare find in a remote village in Wales. If you're serious, you'll just keep looking. An expert in porcelain at Christie's told me he found some plates worth tens of thousands of pounds in a box stuffed at the back of a cupboard under the stairs of a crumbling cottage.

Bargains in antique shops are hard to find, as the dealers tend to know what they're talking about and will price accordingly. But don't be afraid to haggle. According to my sources, the clever trick is to look for 'brown' furniture – Georgian dark wood pieces that are currently unfashionable but bound to come back round again – that you will be able to sell on at a profit (if you're patient). Make sure they're half-decent looking and haven't been badly restored with brown felt-tip pen covering up scratches on the corners. If it looks like tat now, it will still look like tat in 20 years.

Don't hang about in the main area of the shop either. The best finds are in the basement, piled up in the yard at the back or nestling in the cobwebbed corner. Good dealers will always be happy to help you if you're a keen learner, although they do get a bit impatient with time-waster window shoppers. To keep the price down, offer to pay in cash and be prepared to carry the stuff home yourself. After all that, have a nice bit of cake in the olde tea shoppe next door. There's always one next door, in the country.

DO

Chat to the antique shop owner about the origins of a piece you're interested in.

Seek out unfashionable pieces – like legwarmers and ra-ra skirts, they're bound to come back into favour again later.

Take plenty of cash for a quick sale.

DON'T

Haggle for a delightful chest of drawers and chop it up for firewood as soon as you get it out of the shop.

5

Gold Ropes

Visiting Stately Homes

In the countryside there's one sure way to know when spring has arrived. Not when the birds are singing all the day long or the sun puts its hat on, but when the stately homes of England throw open their doors for paying visitors. Opening up again after winter, that halcyon time when they dance naked behind the gold ropes or whatever they're inclined to do when out of sight, they're after some cold cash – to cover the cost of those gold ropes, or just the heating bill.

While some are still owned by the original families, the vast majority of ticketed stately homes are owned by the National Trust, which are visited by 100 million people every year. You don't have to go too far to seek out these grand bastions with their echoes of a past world. Within an hour or so of London you can find the medieval castle, Bodiam; Claydon House, a mansion with rococo furnishings better than anything Laurence Llewelyn-Bowen could hope to muster in a lifetime; and even a little-known collection of Turner paintings at Petworth House. From Birmingham, you can seek out a Tudor manor, Packwood House, with a seventeenth-century yew garden that is supposed to represent the 'Sermon on the Mount'. Or if Doncaster is your starting point, go to Nostell Priory, with its glorious Robert Adam interiors.

The National Trust, which is not without its detractors, has saved thousands of houses around Britain by taking over the running costs when the gentry can no longer afford it themselves. In exchange, if they haven't sold up completely, the families may still live there, opening up their home to the public for several months of the year.

So you must take care when visiting these houses as some of them still have private living quarters. If you go to the magnificent Petworth House, for example, be sure not to go through a door marked 'Private' as you may startle Lord Egremont or one of his family as they go about their daily lives. Despite the size of the place, most families in a National Trust house live squashed into a couple of rooms and a kitchen: more council estate than private estate.

Country people are snobs about stately homes. If they are not National Trust property, the creaking, ancient house will drain a family of all its money and the gentrified inhabitants are required to be the servants of their own home in ways that their ancestors never were – running tea rooms, hosting weddings, pruning the roses and checking in the coats. Those that live in the surrounding village and know the family well will never tire of boasting of the fact, recounting at every opportunity that 'I just popped into Bucketload Hall – well, let me tell you, Tiggles simply can't function without my fairy cakes for the Sad Children's Tea Party'. But the worst snobs are those who live within spitting distance of the grand house but have never had an invitation to get in without paying for the privilege. To them, of course, Bucketload Hall is an absolute disgrace and the best thing for the village would be to repurpose it as a five-star hotel, which everyone could use.

Whether you approve or not of small families living in large houses, contained within the bricks and mortar are stories of war, romance, royalty and pillaging. The volunteers who work there may not always be period historians but they will be enthusiastic and keen to answer questions. And look out for the portraits whose eyes follow you around the room...

DO

Treat these houses with respect: they are fragile and beautiful and only survive because of careful conservation.

Ask if this is a Humphry Repton garden – it may well be and you are bound to impress the guide.

Leave the scissors at home – don't take any cuttings for your own garden.

DON'T

Go if you know the family that lives there – how embarrassing to bump into them from the wrong side of the rope.

5

Wild Times

Badger spotting

Stress. That's the thing about living in a city. You run for the train, your mobile is permanently clamped to your ear, you write endless to-do lists, suffer from road rage, cashpoint rage and Oyster Card rage (if you live in the capital): you don't always know what you've got to do, you just know you've got to get on with it.

Not in the country. It's the lack of urgency that can take you by surprise every time you get out of the Big Smoke – and there is little that requires less urgency than badger watching.

Townies, with their central heating and minimal exposure to the outside air, are not generally suited to wildlife watching. Rather than sit for several hours, stock still, hardly breathing, in order to catch a glimpse of a lesser-spotted wotsit, we would rather leave all that to David Attenborough and watch the edited highlights.

But there are rewards in doing it for real – especially if you do it the townie way: with a five-star bedroom and a deep-tissue massage waiting for you at the end of it.

The only serious attempt I've made at wildlife watching was in the grounds of a grand hotel in Wetherby, Yorkshire. The private woods contained one of the largest badger setts in the North – six different setts, totalling approximately 170 of the black-and-white snouty nosed creatures. The gamekeeper had walked the woods for 30 years and knew every twig and nest in there. We marched into the darkening wood; like many embedded countrymen, he was a man of few words. We just listened to the sounds of the wildlife around us.

Badgers are a rather contentious issue for countrymen. They have been blamed for the spread of TB, and they cause numerous road accidents: out of a population of 300,000, around 50,000 are killed on the roads every year.

The setts are quite easy to spot – the female badgers are very houseproud, and all the paths to their home are swept and tidy. We walked for 20 minutes or so to the depths of the woods, until we found an entrance: a hole leading underground, covered in leaves. We threw out some peanuts and raisins (in the summer badgers like slices of melon) and sat back and waited. The sun got lower, the air got colder, our breath was held. Little whispers were exchanged, as the gamekeeper alerted us to the call of a pheasant or the flight of a crow. But mostly we sat there with heightened anticipation (and not a lot of action). We didn't actually see a badger in the three hours we were out there. But, hey, we knew we were looking at where they lived and we were breathing the same air. For our guide, and even for us, that was enough. Although I couldn't help feeling a little jealous when I was told that the lucky couple who had been taken out the week before saw 12 in one night.

DO

Wear dark clothing and avoid spraying yourself liberally with Chanel No. 5.

Be prepared to sit for hours in the freezing cold without spotting your prey.

Book a spa treatment for the evening – your muscles will ache from sitting still for a long time.

DON'T

Kidnap the badgers and try to sell them to the local zoo.

6

Shopping and Jumping

Badminton Horse Trials

Townies get the opportunity to gather *en masse* all the time – whether at a rave, a May Day riot or just the rush hour. But country people wait for a few big events to come round each year, each of which signals a jolly crowd scene. The first of these, usually in early May, is the Badminton Horse Trials – or, as regulars call it, Badminton.

Just off the M4 in Gloucestershire, nearly 200,000 rural types will converge to watch a cross-country horse race, go shopping and see their mates. Of all the country gatherings, this is the thoroughbred event. What with all those horses and toffs meeting up, there's an awful lot of braying.

There was a lot of heated excitement one year when the popular royal Zara Phillips – an accomplished eventer, holding the British and World titles, as well as the BBC's *Sports Personality of the Year* – planned to compete there on her favourite horse, Toytown. As a four-star event, a good result at Badminton can secure a place in the British team for the Olympics. Unfortunately she had to pull out at the last minute: the tension was as great as Beckham breaking a metatarsal bone in his foot just before the World Cup. Straining at the bit beside her is the horse world's (possibly only) sex symbol, William Fox-Pitt, on Ballincoola. These two are currently our British stars and the ones you must cheer most enthusiastically as they gallop past.

Before you go tearing off with banners and capacious shopping bags, here is the lowdown. The event is held in the Duke of Beaufort's parkland, which is green, manicured and very beautiful. The crowd, however, is not. Dirt under the fingernails and green wellies are the only sartorial requirements. Leave the Marc Jacobs wedges and Prada parka at home.

If, however, you have yet to own such wardrobe necessities as a tweed flat cap or gumboots, you can get it all at Badminton. You see, despite the country folk protesting that they love animals and open spaces, really, it's shopping that turns them on, just like the rest of us. Deprived most of the year of any sort of Mecca to consumerism, except for the village shop, at Badminton, with 500 stalls beckoning, they quite understandably go mad. Think of it as a Bluewater for country folk.

When not shopping, shuttlecocks (those who go to Badminton, as I like to call them) can be found following the horses round the cross-country course and pitching up to cheer at certain fences (the lake fence is the most popular). But I recommend that if you don't want to get soaked to the skin don't set up a picnic by the big water jumps. Lots of people there will be showing off their dogs, because, for once, there's a crowd of admirers handy. Even the car park can look like something of a motor show. After all those cold winter months in the country wilderness, it's spring and there's an audience. Give them a round of applause.

DO

Try to sit by the lake fence – the most dramatic jump of the course.

Take your dog – as preened as a Crufts entrant.

Take your wallet – as full as possible.

Use the main scoreboard as a meeting place.

DON'T

Set up a French cricket game next to the jumps.

7

Leave the Eyebrows Alone

Stag Weekends

Stag weekends – it's never just a night, now, is it? – are steadily growing in expense and bravura. Perhaps friends don't get together enough, perhaps the idea of marriage as a ball and chain to a wild rover's existence has taken a stronger hold and requires a bigger send-off, or perhaps we work harder so the need to let off steam is more overwhelming. But there's no question that for the male, the opportunity for some physical bonding and bragging holds allure and there is no better place for it than in the wide open spaces of the countryside.

Not to mention that, for the nervous fiancée, a stag party away from the city centres, with their high ratio of laptop dancers to drunk men, can only appeal. The nearest rival in the mudlands will only be Dolly the sheep. For men, the countryside provides the best chance to *be* men – you know, paintballing each other, or downing 12 pints of real ale.

If the weather is up to it, I would recommend

camping (see chapter 10). First off, you have the excuse to stay sober until at least the hour when the tents are erected. As one stag event company's website puts it: you don't want to be wandering about by 8.30 p.m. saying your name is Susan. Second, any drunken damage will only occur to your own property. Third, if you choose a quiet camping spot, you will be miles from anyone else and can sing your favourite football and rugby songs long and loud until you collapse in a quivering heap by the dying embers of the fire. Fourth, there is no chance of getting into a fight outside the kebab shop at 5.30 a.m. Finally, there are plenty of butch jobs to do: collect wood for the fire, spitroast the suckling pig (*not* another name for a footballer's WAG), eat baked beans from a tin and so on.

For more comfort, book a house to stay in – as far as possible from any neighbours. In all honesty, you should probably 'fess up in advance that you are a stag party – but be warned, they may then refuse the booking. Collect deposits from everyone early on and work on the basis that you may not get it back. But to minimise damage: lots of water, orange juice, bacon, bread, cheese, milk, coffee and painkillers should be stocked up first. Organise a strenuous activity during the day, which requires sobriety – go-karting, paintballing, clay pigeon shooting, archery, golf – and order a takeaway for your return to the house. Check the local pub in advance – a quiet country pub more used to the patronage of Old Macdonald and his collie is not going to welcome a marauding group of townies braying and banging the tables.

As with the hen weekends (see chapter 8), remember to book taxis in advance; stock up well as the nearest shops are not only going to be miles away but may shut after 4 p.m. on Saturday; take cash not credit cards (to limit your spending and also prevent any damaging losses), and clean up behind you.

DO

Stock up on hangover cures well in advance – the village shop probably won't be open on Sunday morning.

Encourage manly activities: making fires, climbing, mountain biking.

Go camping – the butch version – and you can make as much noise as you like.

DON'T

Take your credit card – cash will limit the amount you can spend on flaming sambucca shots.

Shave off the groom's eyebrows.

8

Clucktastic

Hen Weekends

It's a funny thing but despite the vast number a girl attends in a lifetime, you never hear one say: 'I'm going on a hen weekend... I'm *so* looking forward to it.' But there is an alternative. Instead of spending your hard-earned cash and precious free time drinking overpriced alcopops out of willy-shaped straws in a nightclub, plan your next hen weekend in the countryside.

The great advantage of a hen weekend in a rural setting is that there is no chance of bumping into your boss/aunt/boyfriend just as you are about to launch into a vodka-fuelled Beyoncé-style dance routine at the bus-stop. In a rented house with no neighbours the music can be turned up as loud as you like and go on for as late as you like. Even better, when you're not in a hotel there aren't other guests complaining to the manager about the 4 a.m. renditions of 'She'll Be Coming Round the Mountain'.

Something about being in the middle of nowhere seems to make people lose their inhibitions in a way

28

that they wouldn't in a restaurant: the best 'truth or dare' games are played in a cottage in Exmoor. If you go to the local nightspot, the DJ will give you shout-outs all night, the local boys will be thrilled to see you and if you lose your purse in the back of the cab on the way home, the driver will probably deliver it back to you the next day (that's happened to me!).

A word of caution though. Rented houses are small businesses and the last thing you want to do is ruin it for them by trashing the rooms or scaring the locals. Also, the point of a country hen weekend is to bring some measure of elegance to your demeanour. Don't turn up in a bright pink limo, bang on the village shop door at midnight begging for fags, ask for directions to the kebab shop (there isn't one), demand that the vicar joins in or request a drum 'n' bass medley at the nightclub. Remember that once you are there the nearest shops will be miles away: if possible, load up from a cash 'n' carry on the way for all your drink, food and willy-straw needs.

You will probably have to do a little more planning than usual. But the countryside pursuits available to you are more fun than pedicures: croquet, riding, ping-pong, a hangover-curing long walk. Often the people you rent the house from can organise these for you. Finally, remember to watch out for the cows. No, not the things that stand in fields and moo – the other girls.

DO

Make sure you have ALL your food and drink needs organised in advance.

Book taxis in advance from/to train station and from/to local nightclub.

Remember to pack suitable footwear and warm clothing for the daytime country activities.

DON'T

Bang on the village shop door at midnight, demanding fags and booze.

SUMMER

9

Banger Bargains

Car Boot Sales

The townie booting experience generally takes place in a grimy multi-storey car park and involves rummaging in the back of a Ford Fiesta to yield temptations such as a bag of elastic bands or granny's nightie. These 20 pence bargains then sit in your flat gathering more dust until you finally chuck them where they should have gone in the first place: in the bin. But what of the car boots of yore? Where rare antiques and original fifties teasets are found nestling between the spare tyre and the back window? I can't promise anything to change your fortune, but the place to go for slightly-better-than-tat treasures is the countryside. Booting here falls into two camps: the stately home car boot sale, and the weekly event in the county town.

Of the first, the country house car boot sale is the booter enthusiast's Holy Grail. These run over the summer months and raise money for charity. Booters are invite-only, ensuring that, as a buyer, you don't mistakenly deal in stolen goods or pay hard-earned cash for an overpriced 'antique' from a dealer. Here you will find Lady Toff's chintz cushions and Lord Fop's cigar box. Some stuff will be a (legal) steal, some will cost you more; but then, for £50, you might end up with a kitchen table for your flat that is more used to the attendance of butlers than last night's takeaway curry. Such is the draw of picking at posh rejects, even A-listers are attracted. In the past, the likes of Stella McCartney and Gwyneth Paltrow have given their cast-offs to a car boot. But just like Privilege car insurance, you don't have to be posh to get it. For the price of the £5 entry fee, one day, my son, all this could be yours...

Of the more typical car boot sales, the trick is to pick the right county. Just as the best vintage (remember when they were called 'second-hand'?) clothes are found in charity shops where the locals are rich and therefore likely to be chucking out good stuff, such as Edinburgh's New Town and London's Islington, the best booting is to be found in the richer counties, such as Berkshire, Hampshire and Sussex. Get there early for first dibs, although if you can hang about until the end of the day, there are bargains to be had when sellers just want to get rid of their load. Don't forget to take cash and carrier bags (don't take plastic bags to country car booters: you will be frowned upon for your lack of green awareness). And haggling in the country is fine: after all, that's the fun of the fair.

DO

Haggle – that's the point of car booting, the sellers will only be disappointed if you don't.

Take masses of change for better cash negotiations.

Get there early for first viewing or late for end-of-the-day bargains.

DON'T

Try to buy anything sitting on the driver's seat of the car, or anything the seller is actually wearing.

10

Spit at Stars

Camping

A spot of sunshine brings a spring to everyone's step. In town, the bottled tan can at last be topped up by the real thing. In the country, they carry on camping. This doesn't mean the farmers start mincing in the farmyard and asking Dale Winton down for the weekend; it really is all about getting the tents out.

You would think that breathing clean air all the time, smelling the freshly cut grass each morning and identifying the tunes of 43 different bird songs would be quite enough of the outdoors for anyone, but country folk just can't get enough of it. During the summer months, rustic friends of mine will barely sleep under the roof they slave to pay for, as each weekend is spent out in the back garden with their children. And one Lord I know, in Suffolk, will put up summer guests not in one of his numerous bedrooms but out on the estate under a patched up canvas awning that has been passed down the family generations for almost as long as the silver. But before you head off to join in, be aware that they don't camp it up in the country like the townies do.

First off, people in the country don't use stylish tents (such as those by Cath Kidston, or a paint-your-own tent from art shops), in much the same way that they avoid prettily patterned wellies. Instead, they prefer ex-army tents (all the better if grandpa had used it during the war), or failing that, something in plain green from Milletts. Don't be surprised if they just stick four poles in the ground and drape an oil cloth over the top. This is partly because they don't want to be pretentious, and partly because they want to be camouflaged, to encourage the wildlife to get closer. The only other necessary kit is a sleeping bag, bin bag, matches, torch, Swiss army knife, old saucepan, can of baked beans, bread, milk and teabags. There's no gourmet cooking on a rural camp, just beans on toast.

Next, the site. Most countrymen simply camp out in their gardens (which do tend to average out at the size of a small London park, after all). If they go further afield, it will most likely be to their friend's fields. You can do the same: just make sure you get permission from the farmer first, before banging in the pegs. You will also need to double-check with the site owner before lighting a camp fire – but it's best if you can go somewhere that specifically allows this. Anyone in the country who camps says it's the fire that makes it all worthwhile; learn some traditional folk songs to sing round it, and enjoy the strange sensation of a wet bottom and hot face at the same time. Finally, remember that in a farmer's field you won't have a bathroom.

Although I shouldn't recommend this, the fact is that country folk simply relish peeing in the bushes and not bothering to wash for a few days. You see, they live there because they genuinely love it – the wilds, the wildlife, the damp. And camping is the perfect way to get down and dirty. Ooh, missus.

DO

Be a soil-muncher – sleep under the most basic awning you can find.

Get down and dirty with your co-camper – pee in the bushes and don't wash if you can help it.

Expect to be shown your 'room' on the lawn when staying with a Lord of the Manor.

DON'T

Cook anything you haven't killed unless it comes from a tin.

Sleep indoors at all from May to September.

Forget to camouflage up.

Camp in the bull field.

11

Hook, Line and Sinker

Fishing

In every life a little rain must fall and in Britain our lives are waterlogged. For townies, a rainy day merely means drinking indoors rather than out in the beer garden. But country folk cheer: it's the perfect weather for fishing, especially in the summer. When the May flies are hatching on the river, the trout are sent into spasms of delight and a country fisherman I know describes the normally calm riverside scenes as 'carnage' as men grab their rods and run to the waters.

But don't go digging up a few worms from the garden and rushing out of the door in a bid to catch your tasty and healthy supper. There's a whole world of rules when it comes to fishing in the lakes, rivers and quarries of the great outdoors.

Before you do anything at all you need to get a National Rod Licence (short term or annual). Who knew rods could be so thrillingly illicit? Do you think the gangs of south London could be enticed to fight with them instead of guns, if they knew they could still have the high of owning something without a licence? Anyway – rather un-sexily – you can get these from the local post office or online (see Directory).

Next, you need to decide whether you want to be a coarse angler or a fly-fisher. It's not to do with how much you swear (although it is hard to imagine that Gordon Ramsay could be anything other than a coarse angler when he holds his rod). In the words of Tim Knight, editor of *Angler's Mail*, 'Coarse fishing is where you put things back gently rather than take them home to eat, and you use baits that smell, i.e. maggots. The fly-fisher keeps his catch and uses bits of fluff for bait.' Coarse anglers mainly catch carp, grayling or pike; fly-fishers catch trout and salmon.

The best way to remember it is that on the whole fly-fishers catch fish you'd want to eat, coarse anglers don't, which is why they throw their fish back in, I guess. Valentine Warner, chef and keen angler, told me a recipe for grayling. Gut the fish and lay it on a wooden board, well seasoned with salt, pepper and lemon. Put in a hot oven for 30 minutes. Remove from the oven, chuck the fish and eat the board.

Allegedly, the best way to tie your feather to the hook is with your girlfriend's pubic hair. The pheromones work magic in attracting the fish. If these fishermen sound weird, I wouldn't worry about them too much – at least they've *got* girlfriends. This is a genuine question from an early edition of Trivial Pursuit: What kind of fisherman keeps worms in the fridge? A divorced one.

To look the part, you need to wear tweed and waders

if you go fly-fishing and camouflage gear for baiting carp and grayling. But you don't have to stick to one or the other – basically if you want to catch and eat your trout, you go fly-fishing. But if you want to kiss the carp (I'm told country fishermen kiss fish more frequently than they kiss their wives) and put it back in the water, you get the maggots out. Countrymen do both – it depends on the river and the time of year as to which is best.

But the thing to know is that fishing is not really about the fish. Hours and hours pass by without anything biting your hook: this leaves plenty of time to stare at the water, or the other bank, or just doze. While you might get competitions set up along canals in London, in the country it's about sitting in silence. Serious country fishermen set up bivvies (sort of pop-up tents, presumably derived from bivouacs) which mean they can stay by the riverbank for days on end. Seriously. They may be fishing all night long, or at least sleeping with a toe tied to the line, just in case. If you have spent hours, or even days fishing, you don't want to miss a single catch.

Finally, fishing is not a sociable sport. If you go fishing, even with your very best friend and especially if you go with someone you don't know, remember not to talk to each other all day long.

DO

Pinch a pube from your girlfriend for your bait.

Form a gangsta persona if you plan on fishing without a licence.

Wear tweed for fly-fishing; camouflage gear for coarse angling.

DON'T

Talk to any of your fishing companions.

Forget to pack a flask of whisky – the days can be long and cold.

Play your favourite rap at full ghetto-blast on the riverbank.

12

Tea with the Queen

Royal Ascot Week

For big hats and big bets there's only one event in the calendar that counts: Royal Ascot Week. Even HM The Queen gets excited about Ascot, hosting a house party at Windsor Castle for the full four days. If you want to check out her latest pastel-coloured suit and hat, make sure you get there in time for the daily royal procession at 2 p.m.

Like the Grand National, Ascot has appeal even for those who don't normally bet on the gee-gees. There are several races every day from Tuesday to Friday (and some new ones on Saturday, too), and the world's top jockeys and horses will be there. Excitement is also generated by the fact that it is still what people think of when they think of 'the Season', the summer round-up of jollies that the toffs would unfailingly attend every year. Few can spare the time and money to do that now, but Ascot remains a key summer event if you want to see and be seen.

Of course, it's not just anywhere on the Ascot

racecourse that you want to be spotted – it's in the Royal Enclosure. This area is the one that generates the heat. The entrance to this is jealously guarded by stewards in green bowlers, and adherence to the rules is strict: if you have not been invited to the Royal Enclosure, you're not coming in. No matter *who* you are – as Joan Collins discovered to her embarrassment one year. To be invited is a fairly archaic process – you have to be nominated by an existing member who has attended the race meeting for at least four years. When I first went (naturally to the Royal Enclosure), I do remember finding it astonishing that such divisions – which were, in all honesty, largely about class – could still have such tangible reality, particularly after the landslide victory of the Labour government in 1997. And it appears that such divisions are, in fact, becoming ever harder to maintain (yay!).

Following a recent extensive modernisation, significant changes have been made to the racecourse and the stands. For one thing, the division between the Royal Enclosure and everywhere else is not as apparent as it once was. For many toffs, this makes the whole day out much less interesting – it was rarely about the horses and more about bumping into your friends – and many have stopped going. I suspect Ascot will become a much less posh affair, but the appeal of dressing up and outlandish hats will remain.

Wander around close to the Royal Enclosure, where most of the corporate boxes are, and you should get up close and personal with several top toffs and a smattering of the smarter celebrities and minor royals.

There's a nice little illustration here, too, of the British attitudes to snobbery. If you look up into the stands of the Royal Enclosure you'll notice that all the men keep their top hats on – except for one small section, where they are bareheaded. These men are in the Royal Box and a slight change of the rules ensures their higher status is on display for all to see. Snobbery is really about getting into a box within a box.

The Royal Enclosure is the only place where you are obliged to adhere to a strict dress code (morning suit and top hat for the men; trouser or dress suit and a hat covering the crown of the head for the women), but it wouldn't really be Ascot if you didn't take pleasure in wearing a hat wherever you stand – the bigger and more outrageous, the better. The best day for the extreme hat parade is Gold Cup Day, otherwise known as 'Ladies' Day', on the Thursday. If you want to get your picture in the papers, this is the day to try. Gold Cup Day is also traditionally the day of the best races: in fact, for all the high society frippery, Ascot has superb racing, with millions given away in prize money over the five days.

So don't forget to place your bets. Buy a race card and put a quid each way on as many horses as you can afford; the atmosphere of the huge crowd cheering on a sunny day is England at both its best ... and its worst.

DO

Wear a big hat.

Take the train – traffic is awful and the car parks are full of regulars, making it nigh on impossible to find a space.

Try to get invited to a car park picnic – some people bring their own butlers.

Buy a race card and place a bet.

Keep your top hat on in the Royal Enclosure – unless you are in the Royal Box.

DON'T

Try to make your own Royal Enclosure badge, *Blue Peter*-style, and hope the stewards won't notice – you'll be thrown out faster than a horse bolts the starter gate.

13

Never Play by the Rules

Croquet

So it rains in August. 'So what?' say the yokels. Townies need to make like country folk and pretend the weather doesn't matter when it comes to summer fun. In the hinterlands they're quite mystified as to how 'rain stops play'. So to get you off your behinds, here's countryside summer sport, with the unwritten rules writ down for you right here.

The quintessential country game is surprisingly deadly – it nearly ended one prominent minister's career when he was spotted playing it one summer: croquet. In any country house you are sure to find a coffin-shaped battered wooden box with mallets heavier than anything used by a circus strongman and coloured hoops with vicious pointy ends. Despite the political ignominy and dangerous tools, countrymen – and women – swear by croquet as the ultimate pulling tool. If the host is trying to get you into the bedroom later, then chances are you will find that there is much encouragement to 'smack the balls harder' and play

47

through hoops set behind the shrubbery to encourage amorous desires.

The first difficulty for any guest playing croquet is that, while there are official rules, in any given private garden you will be expected to play to 'house rules'. And of course, they often won't reveal these rules until after you have broken them (touching the flower-bed means you miss a go, for example). But don't worry too much. A Wiltshire player tells me that everyone should 'cheat like hell' for it to be any fun at all. The main thing about cheating at croquet is that it is deemed to be OK, so long as you are not caught in the act. One good house trick, favoured by the late Lord Wyatt of Weeford, was to declare: 'Here we play the Crichton-Michael convention: bisques at six and eight, all roquets taken by the strike.' This actually meant nothing at all, but the guests would be too embarrassed to admit their ignorance, leaving the host free to make up the rules as he went along, so he could win.

Auberon Waugh would allow women and clergymen to play to different rules from the rest. Another trick is to do a mincing walk between two hoops: this both distracts the other player and creates a shallow channel in the lawn for the ball to easily slide down and through the hoop.

Play in teams and you will find good camaraderie in the subterfuge. But don't expect a quiet game – every game of croquet ends in chaos, with guests shouting that they weren't told about the hidden bumps and slopes in the playing field and dogs madly trying to chase the wooden balls.

Some top cheats, as suggested by the editor of *The Field*, Jonathan Young: after a bad shot, scream loudly that you've been stung by a wasp – you'll get to play your move again; don't stick to your own ball – just play the most convenient one; trip on hoops that are getting in your way and move them somewhere more to your advantage; spike the Pimm's.

The object is to get really hot and sweaty and in need of a good long glass of homemade lemonade afterwards. And if the croquet doesn't get you going, just ask a countryman to help you out: he'll have his way.

Basic Rules of Garden Croquet:

To be played with six hoops and four balls, with two balls on each side. Object of the game: to advance the balls around the lawn by hitting them with a mallet, scoring a point for each hoop made in the correct order and direction. Winning side is first to score the six hoop points and one peg point per ball (after you've been through all the hoops, you have to hit the peg at the end). Players take turns and only one plays at a time.

Earn extra shots by scoring the next hoop in order or by striking your ball so that it hits one of the other balls (earns two extra shots).

DO

Cheat like hell and make up the rules as you go along, especially if the game is taking place in your own garden.

Use the game as a pulling tool – amorous inclinations are often unleashed in the heart of the action.

Expect a little tactical subterfuge – croquet is a serious business!

DON'T

Suggest the coffin-shaped box the hoops and mallets are kept in is used to bury the next small pet that dies.

14

A Fête Accompli

Village Fêtes

In the summertime, there is one quintessentially countryside event that everyone thinks must be too idyllic to be true, but in fact still goes on: the village fête. Usually held to raise money for the church steeple or the children's playground, these are local affairs and one of the loveliest ways to enjoy the countryside at its very best.

Practically every village hosts its own fête in its own special way, but whichever one you go to, there is a country code to follow for all. The best way to find one is simply to take a drive out to the countryside on any given weekend during the more balmy time of year and look out for hand-painted signs announcing the festivities. Choose a sunny day, wear your most casual country clothes (wellies, corduroys, moth-eaten shirt) and take plenty of small change. These are the very last places in the world where you can pick up a cake, jigsaw or tomato plant for less than a quid.

There are certain types you can always spot at a fête.

The organiser will usually be a large-bosomed, bossy woman, a proud member of all the local committees and generally spotted in church every Saturday morning, overseeing the flower arrangements. At the fête, you'll see her inspecting all the stalls, rallying the villagers to buy raffle tickets and prodding the sponge cakes to make sure they're genuinely home-made. The vicar will stroll about, batting off his housewife fans and exhorting the men to take part in the 'rat-catcher' game (a bundle of fake fur chucked down a chute that you have to hit with a mallet at the bottom) for 50p a go. Pushy-dad will also be there, telling his children not to whine but grin and bear it in the stocks, as everyone chucks wet sponges at them.

Some fêtes are brilliantly imaginative, displaying British humour at its best. The Harting village fête in Sussex features a human fruit machine, where you hand over your coins, and three men turn round and pick a piece of fruit from a basket. If all three choose the same one, you win a prize. Have a go on hook-a-duck, get your face painted, have a chance at the lucky dip or take a shot at the coconut shy. Pleasures you thought went out with the steam train will suddenly take on more appeal than anything a PlayStation could do. You'll get sick on gallons of tea, rounds of fairy cakes, wodges of candyfloss and home-made lemonade, stickier than a fly-catcher. Some fêtes tug on the nostalgic heartstrings with period themes, such as the 1940s at the Radley village fête and flower show, or the more elaborate eighteenth-century staging of the Milton Abbas fête in Dorset.

But you don't always need to look to the past. At the Tillington fête in West Sussex, you can go bell-ringing on Saturday and on Sunday sip Pimm's by the village cricket match, with an evening picnic and fireworks. Sometimes, just sometimes, there's nothing better than a classic British summer's day.

DO

Have a go – at everything on offer – come on, you only live once!

Donate – fêtes raise money for local causes, so be generous on the cake stall.

Take your manners with you – it's an old-fashioned event and requires a gentle approach.

DON'T

Expect any fairground rides or even anything that requires a battery.

Cry if you lose at the raffle – the tickets are probably only 10p each anyway.

15

Gonna Get Married

Country weddings

You know that tedious time of year: all your money is drained on pointless presents and party outfits you wouldn't normally wear in your own back garden, let alone in public. Not Christmas – the wedding season. The best of these take place in the countryside: the country house setting is the Holy Grail of all romantic couples, just think Jordan and Peter, Madonna and Guy, Posh and Becks, Paul McCartney and Heather Mills – OK, perhaps the least said about that particular union, the better. One year, in a single summer's weekend, four footballers married their WAGs in four of Britain's grandest stately homes. But if you've been invited to one, you need to know the rules – not the offside one, the real country code.

There are two types of country wedding. First, the one where townies hire the biggest stately home they can find (many a crumbling pile has been rescued in this way); these tend to be all about the bling, with hundreds of guests vying for a picture in *Hello*! The second type is for the country-dwellers, where the wedding ceremony takes place in a village church and the reception is held in their parents' back garden. But, whichever one you're going to, certain rules apply to all.

First off, book your B&B. Don't assume that because the wedding is at Blenheim Palace you will be staying there – millionaire footballer John Terry recommended his guests stay at the local £60 a night Peartree Travelodge hotel. Try and find one that has a bar and might consider a lock-in scenario for whisky drinking with fellow revellers. And make sure they will serve you breakfast beyond 9 a.m. Next, book your cab from the reception to the B&B. There will inevitably be only three local cabs available to ferry 250 guests around.

Next, within a week of receiving the invitation you should buy the present from the wedding list, usually sent with the invitation. (Posh brides get their list at John Lewis, the less pretentious will go to Argos.) This should ensure that you are not left buying the only remaining presents such as the £95 pepper grinder or an ironing board.

When planning your outfit, remember that you can always rely on the presence of a fresh country breeze, so don't wear a hat with too large a brim. Stilettos will always sink into the grass, too, but I still prefer height to flat shoes: just pick the mud off before going into the marquee. It helps to remember to pack your outfit in the first place, too. I once drove at high speed, late as usual, to the B&B I was staying at for a grand wedding in Wiltshire. As I ran up the stairs to my room for a quick change, I suddenly stopped halfway. I had brought my hat, shoes and my bag. My carefully dry-cleaned outfit was still lying on the bed in London. I had to go in what I was wearing: a cheap cotton skirt from New Look and a camisole-style top. I wore the (utterly unmatching) hat anyway and apologised profusely to the bride's mother: 'I wondered why you were in a thermal vest,' she sniffed.

Get to the church early. This isn't to bag your pew but to talk to the villagers hanging around outside, gawping (and laughing) at the townies. If you don't want to end up on the local website for the caption of the week competition, be nice to them. Village churches tend to be on the small side, and you're likely to be in a scrum at the back – but this is usually a good opportunity to check out the potential dance partners for later. Be wary of offering your shoulder where it's not needed though – the problem with weddings in the country is that you can't tell whether someone is being emotional or just has really bad hayfever.

In the country, everyone gets bussed over to the reception – don't miss it or you could find yourself walking several lonely miles while everyone is tucking into champagne and cake. If you're driving, there will usually be a field allocated as a car park, but that doesn't necessarily mean they've cleaned the cow pats out, so watch your step.

The reception is where the country wedding really comes into its own. All those dark bushes outside, not to mention the tens of bedrooms lying tantalisingly empty in the big house and all of you miles and miles from anywhere. Apparently more couples hook up at weddings than anywhere else – I blame the champagne goggles and the flattering cut of the morning suit or the carefully chosen dress. Be careful out there.

DO

Check the B&B has a bar so you can carry on the party.

Book your cab weeks in advance.

Be nice to the villagers who turn up to watch the guests arrive.

Be prepared to sit next to the vicar, or his wife, at the dinner.

DON'T

Miss the bus taking you to the reception because you've started snogging in the church graveyard.

Try and find a present that is not on the list. They don't want it: that is why it isn't on the list.

16

The Sport of Kings

Polo

High-octane glamour isn't just for town. In fact, in June and July, during the posh polo season, there will be more champagne, fast cars, tight-trousered men, tanned women and wads of newly minted cash in the countryside than anything you'd ever find at Chinawhite. (Of course, even Chinawhite moves to the country for polo-clubbing.)

Late July is the traditional time for the Veuve Clicquot Gold Cup Final at Cowdray Park in Sussex. Always a popular spot for polo – the late Viscount Cowdray revived the sport there after World War II – this event sees its largest crowd of the year, as the players and their fans descend. This is the more genteel and old-fashioned polo event; the celebrities here will be sportsmen and newsreaders. The best name to drop is Adolfo Cambiaso – an Argentinian; he is to polo what David Beckham is to football. To fit in, wear a linen suit or pretty, but not too revealing, dress.

The following weekend will see a similar scene at

the Cartier International Day at the Guards Polo Club in Windsor – serious polo but much, much more glitzy. There are still some of the old guard here (it's a popular event with the royals) and you will find that they are heavily cordoned off – separating the chavs from the chav-nots. As well as the Queen handing over the prize, you will spot any number of young American TV stars (Mischa Barton and Joshua Jackson being two particularly hot appearances in previous years) mingling over the chukkas. The Z-list soap stars will be there, too, getting drunk on champagne as they picnic by the car park. I've had a high old time in the past drinking myself under the plastic tables on the right side of the white faux-picket fence of the Cartier tent, laughing myself silly at the Russian oligarchs dressed in jodhpurs and boots with nary a polo pony in sight. But there is one democratic event – the treading in of the divots. The ponies' hooves kick up clods of earth during a game, so at half-time it's traditional for the spectators to walk out and stamp them back in.

The ticket everyone wants is for the VIP section of the Chinawhite marquee. It's tacky and cocktail-fuelled but all the A-listers join in. The royal princes will usually be spotted scaling the side of the marquee come midnight, and the wannabe Cinderellas will lose not just their shoes but their knickers too. The essential accessory here is a huge pair of sunglasses and anything with the designer label hanging off the back.

Do try to watch a game or two – polo is known as the other sport of kings. Perhaps because the most handsome, and often rich, men play it. It could also be because watching two teams thunder across the field is said to be the closest we will get to seeing what a cavalry charge must have been like. (And you must try to see when the players swap one pony for another during the game – it's the equestrian equivalent of an F1 pit stop.) Undoubtedly, it is exciting, glamorous and sweaty. More than a mint with a hole can do for you.

NEED TO KNOW:

Polo grounds are 300 yards long and 160 yards wide. Goal posts are 8 yards apart.

The match is divided into chukkas, each lasting seven minutes, with an interval of three minutes between each one. Half-time interval is five minutes.

A bell is rung at the end of each chukka but play continues after the bell until the ball goes out of play. In the final chukka, the bell stops play.

Goal ends are changed after each goal scored or at half-time if there is no score by then.

DO

Dress up: demurely for Cowdray; high-glitz for Cartier.

Stamp in the divots at half-time – even if you're wearing high-heels.

Drop the names Henry Brett and Adolfo Cambiaso – polo's stars.

DON'T

Call the polo ponies 'horses'.

Try to cross the field during a game – it's a race against horsepower.

Ignore the commentary – it brings the match alive.

17

Vinous Ventures

English Vineyards

Townies probably think they've got the edge on binge drinking, with all-night licences and bus-stops to throw up in. But it's out in the country that the stuff is produced – think hops, apples, potatoes and pears – and it's there you can really tuck in.

However, I will grant you, the rural pastime of imbibing used to be somewhat limited to yards of ale, frothy tankards of mead and a killer home-made brew of pear cider. For sophistication, celebration and gustation we would look to our French and New World cousins. Until now.

The increasingly warmer climate of these shores means that the growth and sustainability of English vineyards has reached Gallic proportions. (Which is just how country people like it – they go abroad as little as possible as they miss their houses and animals too much.) So nowadays, if you are going through your own quarter- or mid-life crisis, you can indulge in a full-on *Sideways* experience right here.

But, before you go racing headlong into the countryside armed with a corkscrew and a wineglass, here are a few pointers.

Wine experts now are agreed that the best thing about English vineyards is their relaxed and laid-back atmosphere. Apparently, this is largely to do with the fact that anyone running a vineyard here must be a bit bonkers and on the edge. Either that, or they've been indulging in those potent home-brews.

Vineyard owners are really farmers, and accordingly scruffy – so leave the black tie at home. Your tour will largely take you round the South East, where the soil and weather closely mimic those of France. Do phone ahead – at Ridgeview vineyards in Sussex, you can picnic and see the orchards with ease, but it's still polite to let them know when you're arriving.

The most picturesque vineyard is Breaky Bottom in East Sussex and they will welcome you with open arms, but perhaps not in the middle of their breakfast (the vineyard's house is a home).

The biggest success story of English vineyards recently has been their sparkling wine. The wines are produced according to *méthode champenoise*, but they are not allowed to call it champagne – that privilege is only accorded to wines grown in France's Champagne region. But in blind tastings English sparkling wine has been winning out over French champagne in recent years.

All of the vineyards are geared up to sell you their wares and are happy to talk you through the tastings. Just remember: the French spit, the British swallow. Guzzle away with gusto, but if you are going to drink a lot, it must mean you like it – so buy a case. And don't be pretentious. If you want to describe the wine, you can do it in plain English.

DO

Take a spread to eat al fresco on the vineyard's estates in summer.

Warn them of your arrival.

Buy the wine you've tasted and enjoyed.

Swallow, don't spit.

DON'T

Drink the spittoon of wine, leave drunk and fail to even buy a bottle.

Bring your own.

Indulge in highfalutin wine speak – say what you think without the waffle.

18

We are Sailing

Cowes Week

If you ever pushed a paper boat across a pond as a child, you need to get down to the Isle of Wight in August and see Cowes Week kick off. Now a world-class yachting regatta, the excitement is in the variety of the boats (1,000 boats of nearly 40 different classes) and the mix of amateur and Olympic champion sailors competing together. It doesn't matter if the nearest you've come to being a sailor is drinking rum – follow my rules and you'll take to it like a rubber duck to bathwater.

First off, you need to look right. At Cowes everyone wears the same clothes day and night – shorts, slightly smelly Dubarry boots or deck shoes, faded T-shirts, sailing fleeces, Kaenon sunglasses at all times (hung round your neck), a visor and, for the finishing touch, wash your hair in salt water. Crew and spectators alike get their clothes from Crew Clothing, Fat Face and Murphy & Nye – all of which have stores in Cowes, so you can get kitted out straightaway. But roll in the sand first – you don't want to look too new.

The races start in the morning – the time will be set by the tide – and go on until at least late afternoon on a good, windy day, but usually until early evening. Each race has its own start time, and the races are divided by the class of boat, rather than sailing ability, and all of them are out in the water following their own race routes: it is a spectacular sight. To watch, go to Cowes Parade and sit on the green. There's a real carnival atmosphere with street entertainment all day, commentary blasting on the tannoys and plenty to drink. It's recommended that you take your own picnic as the food is reported to be pretty grim. Keep your eyes peeled and you'll spot a smattering of celebrities having a low-key day out – Jodie Kidd and Jeremy Irons have been spotted doing the sailor's polka. If you want to pull an Olympian sailor, the champs all drink at The Pier View pub, which boasts a great view of the races too. Ask them about their A-sails, swing-keels and whether they got their tides right. (No, me neither, but it'll get their attention.)

Look on Yachting World's website to discover who the brassiest contenders are. To really get a taste for the event, go to the Royal Yacht Squadron for the race starts and stand by the cannons as they go off.

Everyone starts drinking early – as you might expect, the best sailors are drunken ones. Avoid the main beer tent and hang out in Shepherd's Wharf Marina, on the dockside instead. The Sail For Gold pub on Cowes Parade is good for beer with a view. The Cowes Yacht Haven also has a massive bar with live music, and you can finish off with some dodgy dancing at Inferno's nightclub. Cowes is pretty small, so you'll find everything is within stumbling distance. Don't forget the Alka Seltzer. Ahoy!

DO

Wear sailing kit all day and night – whether you're on a boat or not.

Sign up for an hour's free sailing lesson.

Book accommodation well in advance.

Wear suncream if you go on the water – even if it's a grey day.

Watch the fireworks on the final night – hundreds of boats in the water line up to watch, too.

DON'T

Take cans of spinach and try to give them to the sailors unless you are Olive Oyl.

19

We Built This Village on Rock 'n' Roll

Music Festivals

Long weekends, mud and music: bet that makes you think of Glastonbury. But that, my friends, is what the townie does. Country people have music festivals in their own backyards and steer clear of the urban rockers churning up the fields next door.

Still, the country demographic being what it is – middle-aged folks with their kids – the countryman's rock festival is not what you would call hip. More hip replacement. The image that describes it best would be a mass gathering of embarrassing dads dancing.

If you have a hankering for Bryan Ferry – who seems to headline every single countryside rock event – or any of his dodgy-haired cohorts, you can pitch up and start bopping. But not before you've taken note of the rules on how to be a tweed-rocker. You have to forget anything you've heard about wearing maxi dresses and flower-patterned wellies to the music festivals. Dress is strictly for warmth and comfort: wellies (plain green), Barbour jackets, flat cap, large umbrella. If you don't take a chair, take a 'shooting stick' – a sort of pole you stick in the ground that has a little seat on top, which you can get from any good field sports shop (Farlows, Purdeys). There's no sitting cross-legged and swaying at Hatton House, Warwickshire, or the picnic concert at Battle Abbey: you need to set up a trestle table with white tablecloth and chairs. According to my country friends, this stops the dancers barging past you to the front. At other rock concerts people eat if they've got the munchies, but at these events a three-course supper is laid out and consumed while the artists are giving it their all on the stage.

In the summer, rock icons of the late seventies and early eighties strut their tight-trousered stuff across the countryside. Long abandoned are the seedy nightclubs of town. Instead they perform with a backdrop of England's most beautiful stately homes, looking out at an audience dressed in tweed and chinos, with not a punk in sight.

One genial countryman recalls a bemused crowd of red-faced toffs during an Eric Clapton rendition of 'Cocaine'. When people in the country talk about a drop of the hard stuff, they're usually referring to a single-malt whisky. These country rockers behave as if the full-scale live music and lights were little more than a slightly too loud CD in the background. If a rock ballad comes on, it's not lighters that are waved in the air but glasses of vintage brandy. All of which makes one wonder – is it more astonishing that the gentle country way of life proves itself so resilient, or that these musicians are still rocking?

DO

Take a three-course dinner, white tablecloth and trestle table to set up in front of the stage.

Learn the words to Bryan Ferry's biggest hits.

Sway to the music, but don't dance – unless you find the style of embarrassing dads on the disco floor a sexy sight.

DON'T

Wear your best nightclub bling – country rockers look like they're off on a long, hearty walk.

Take chocolate bars and ginger biscuits 'for the munchies'.

Light up a large joint, unless it's beef.

20

Something Novel

Literary Festivals

Are you sitting comfortably? Then I'll begin. A great asset of the countryside is the round of book festivals that take place in the summer months. This is the time for townies to turn the page and immerse themselves in some cultural learning that goes beyond watching a late night programme on BBC2.

The more discerning amongst you may easily name a few Nobel Prize-winning authors that you ache to meet. But these highbrow sounding gatherings are not just for the intelligentsia – these days anyone who is anyone is putting pen to paper. Or at least paying someone to do it for them. Chefs, politicians, actresses, sportsmen – all claiming a way with words and all appearing at these fests.

There is the charming Aldeburgh Literary Festival, homegrown from the local bookshop; the slightly bigger Bath Literature Festival, and the absolutely immense Hay Festival (if Aldeburgh is the local bookshop, Hay is the Waterstone's of the lit fest world). Tickets sell out fast – although you may be able to grab some returns on the day. But don't be fooled by the quaint tea shops and mild-mannered locals. Devotees of these festivals will put up a fight to see their favourite authors: one year someone stormed the hall in Aldeburgh in an attempt to get a seat to a reading.

These events are largely attended by locals and their friends, but the larger festivals – such as 'the Hay', as it is known by regulars – attract audiences from all over.

Hay is for the big hitters – this otherwise sleepy town in the shadow of the Black Hills becomes a whirlwind of people for nine days in the summer. It's Glastonbury without the high walls and photo ID cards. There are more second-hand bookshops per square mile than anywhere else in the country. So, as with Glastonbury, even if you never manage to get to the main stages, you'll have a great time seeking out the tiny ad hoc events that spring up. Spend all your cash on books – a signed hardback by an unknown now could turn out to be the J.K. Rowling of the future.

To fit in, dress like an academic don at university (I believe 'shabby chic' just about coins it) and swot up on the author beforehand. The standard of questions is generally high and you won't earn any points for asking whether the author prefers Jilly Cooper or Jackie Collins to read on the beach. Don't take every single battered paperback you own by the writer and ask them to inscribe dedications to all the members of your family – just buy the latest work. If you get two or three copies, that will buy you the time in which to declare your undying devotion.

While you will get the odd highbrow reading, there are also informal signings with an author, workshops on how to tap into your own creative flow, poetry slams for teenagers and a lot of wandering around in bookshops and cafes just to pick up on the atmosphere. Let the countryside bring out the novel that's in you.

DO

Snap up some unknown authors' tomes and get them to sign for you – you might have discovered the next big thing.

Book your accommodation well in advance – conveniently close hotels and B&Bs are full up months ahead.

Dress like an academic – and try to think of clever questions.

DON'T

Ask David Starkey for his views on the Queen.

Take the entire back catalogue of your favourite author and expect them to sign every one.

Put up too much of a fight to get into your reading – storming the doors is a step too far.

21

Dude, Where's My Surfboard?

Surfing

You may think of people living in the country as straw-munchers rather than surfing dudes. You'd be wrong. Just a few hours from London are the kind of surfer communities you thought only existed in North Shore Hawaii or the set of *Point Break*. If you get yourself in gear quickly enough, you could be with them in 24 hours, riding the waves.

Newquay in Cornwall is generally acknowledged to be the surfer's capital of the UK, with eleven beaches over seven miles of sand. Watergate beach is one of the most beautiful of these, with a kite-surfing school and a Jamie Oliver restaurant. Cornwall isn't big on motorways, and it can take hours to drive there but there are flights to Newquay from most UK airports. Other big local surfer scenes are in Polzeath, North Cornwall, Woolacombe and Croyde Bay in North Devon and Sennen Cove by Land's End. Nearer to London is West Wittering on the south coast (less than 90 minutes away) and keen surfers will just go where the conditions are right – there's nothing to stop you going to Brighton beach, after all.

When a blisteringly hot weekend has been predicted and there's just a slight offshore breeze (when the wind blows seaward from the land), you'll be looking at the perfect surfer's weather. All you need is first to look the part. Local surfers have a permanent tan (so get out the Fake Bake), sun-bleached hair, shapeless, faded baggy shorts and never, ever wear shoes. If you're a hardcore townie, I'd leave your 4x4 at home and remember to order smoothies at the beach shack, not champagne.

Of course, even if it's hot, the water will be damn cold – and early summer is the coldest time of year in the sea, as the sun hasn't been shining long enough to warm it up like a bowl of your granny's pea soup. You need to wear a wetsuit, and it needs to fit properly or it won't keep you warm. Besides which, a badly fitting wetsuit will chafe your salty skin like sandpaper on a soft plum. Don't bother buying one – they're awkward to carry, stink out your bathroom and take ages to dry out. Besides, at about £8 a pop to hire, they won't break your piggy bank. Hiring boards is also more chic: a pro-surfer would rather get a job in the City than be seen with a brand new board.

Next you need to get out on the waves. If you're a beginner have some lessons first. A classic starter mistake, for example, is to hold the board flat in front of you in the water so that even a small wave causes it to smack you in the face. (Been there, got the bloodied nose.) If you're a beginner, do not go ploughing off to

75

where the experts are. Nothing ruins their weekend more than having to stage a rescue.

The aim in surfing is to 'catch' the wave and then 'ride' it all the way back to the beach. If you are close to another, more experienced, surfer DO NOT attempt to catch the wave first, thus exposing yourself to ridicule if you miss it. It is also strictly against surfer etiquette to try to launch yourself on to a wave that someone is already on as it comes towards you.

Avoid conversation. Leave that to the guys that know each other. If another surfer asks if you want to go 'out back', they're not asking you outside for a fight. 'Out back' refers to the point in the water just beyond the break (where the waves break on the rocks is the 'point break'). The be all and end all for surfers is the 'tube' – not the Northern line, the hollow inside a breaking wave. Keep saying 'tube' and 'dude' a lot and you too could be mistaken for a surfer babe.

DO

Look the part.

Take some lessons.

Get a wetsuit that fits. Anything else can prove painful.

Get hip with the surf dude lingo.

Know that 'out back' has nothing to do with the Aussie game parks.

DON'T

Tell anyone you enjoy your desk job.

22

Birdies in the Clubhouse

Golf

Against all expectation, golf has become an acceptable sport. WABs ('wives and birdies') are all over our newspapers flouting their *de trop* outfits during Ryder Cups, in much the same way as WAGs at World Cups. In the days when the game was represented by the likes of Ronnie Corbett and Bruce Forsyth in diamond-patterned tank tops and loud checked trousers, this turnaround seemed as likely as Wayne Rooney teaching an etiquette class.

But now it is not only played by everyone from Grand Prix racing drivers to Catherine Zeta Jones, it is almost (whisper it) hip. The only thing holding golf back from being a fabulous activity for the weekend has been that women – aside from the odd Welsh movie star – have steadfastly resisted its charms. This has largely been to do with the grim, schoolroom atmosphere of the clubhouses. While the men hunkered down in the bunkers, the women were left sipping G&Ts in a room with all the appeal to their femininity of an oily toolbox.

Women: rejoice. Smart clubhouse managers have slowly begun to realise that it's those cunning XX chromosomes that decide the weekend plans. If they were going to exploit the golf fetish of the male, they needed to provide something for the gals too. Now unisex-friendly clubs have started sprouting around the countryside. A good example is the one at Goodwood, Sussex, run by the eminently enterprising and charming Lord March (the pin-up for Aga-chained wives everywhere). Pay-and-play schemes, here and elsewhere, mean that membership fees only a millionaire can normally afford are outmoded. Just a small annual fee, and the purchase of top-up credits throughout the year, have made golf affordable – so there's no excuse not to take your partner along too, and have a slap-up lunch after nine holes. A decent clubhouse now will entertain the waiting WAB with roaring log fires, newspapers and a supply of G&Ts. At Goodwood, there's even a Ralph Lauren outlet, so you can look the part even if you don't want to play (personally, I've always fancied myself as a bit fetching in a pastel tank top).

These new clubhouses are all the more thrilling for their utter lack of snobbery. Membership is designed to be inclusive, while the owners can rest easy that the calm, elegant interiors are likely to inspire manners to match. The rules are those of gentlemen: do not steal each other's balls, do not speed in the buggies, do not suggest a wife swap. Clothes tend to be reasonably smart: trousers and shirts, no jeans. Apparently the single golfing glove in the back pocket does NOT have the same connotations as the Compton Street handkerchief rule, so you can rest easy there. In places such as Stoke Park (where Bridget Jones had her mini-break) or The Grove, there are spas available too, and you don't have to be a girl to enjoy those. In the case of CZJ and hubby, I imagine she's on the course, striking a birdie, while he's enjoying a top-up of youth-enhancing serum.

DO

Take it slowly in the buggies – those bunkers can spring out of nowhere.

Take the game seriously – golfers are very snooty about amateurs on the course.

Enjoy the clubhouse while your partner is driving balls in the rain – spas, log fires and shopping outlets are increasingly common.

DON'T

Worry about putting your glove in your back pocket – it doesn't mean you're a giver rather than receiver. Honest.

23

Waiting for the Fat Lady

Garden Opera

Townies are a little smug sometimes. Outside our smog-heavy cities might be clean air and the smell of freshly cut grass every day; but towns have more sophistication, with theatres and galleries. Urbanites live where the scenes are happening and if a country bumpkin wants to 'catch a show', they have to drive for several hours to see one.

The smugness is rather misplaced. In the country, especially during the summer, there's more culture than Shakespeare himself could shake a stick at. Rural types go mad for country house operas. I'm not talking about toffs singing in the shower. These are professional, small-scale operas performed in gardens. Often the opera company stays in the house for a few nights, and the owner invites friends and locals to come and watch. (One such hostess consequently spends her summers washing fake blood stains out of the cast's costumes.) Tickets are not only affordable but often raise money for charity, and the whole event is staged in beautiful surroundings. But before you go donning your opera cape and roaring up the motorway, you need to know the rules.

Each country house has its own ways and mores, usually depending on the size of the estate. The Glyndebourne opera season is the original – not to mention grandest – of this scene, setting the precedent for many of them, but you don't always have to wear black tie or know your Puccini from your Wagner. Jane Keenan of The Garden Opera Company says that all their operas are sung in English, as they are determined to be as accessible as possible. Jane recommends a Mozart opera if you are a beginner, as they are generally light and comical.

On the whole, these gigs are hosted by two types of country dweller. First is the former hippy, who wants to prove his or her arty credentials, despite the big house and full complement of staff they now employ. The dress code might be black tie, but of the frayed hand-me-down type, or slightly too-long hair and crumpled linen jackets for the men, and hemp skirts for the women. You can find this crowd at Garsington Opera, Longborough, of which Jilly Cooper is a fan, and any of the smaller venues that The Garden Opera Company performs at. Grange Park Opera is smart-hippy: take your cue from the director of the event, the glamorous Wasfi Kani, and drape yourself in layers of Indian silks. Then there are, of course, the serious opera buffs who want to hear the fat lady sing without having to stay in the Big Smoke. They'll insist on crisp black tie and divine long dresses: see them at

Glyndebourne. The crowds picnicking on the lawns during the interval are sometimes more glamorous and dramatic than the opera itself, so you needn't even bother buying a ticket.

DO

Check the dress code before you go – black tie for Glyndebourne; Indian silks for Grange Park.

Try a Mozart opera if you've never been to one before – the heroine is less likely to die of consumption.

Take a hand-held fan – some summer concerts are held in converted barns and can get unbearably hot.

DON'T

Worry if you don't know your Verdi from your Vermicelli – it's as much about the picnic as the opera.

Crack any jokes about plump ladies.

24

Something Fishy

Coastal Gourmet

Townies are chow-down champions when it comes to eating out. In one year 158 new restaurants opened in London alone, leading food-stuffers to declare that current generations are living in a 'Golden Age' of dining. Is the countryside following suit? All those lambs ready for the slaughter and golden fields of corn should bring high hopes. But restaurants are the weakest link when it comes to gourmet delights in England's pleasant lands. The only Michelin you're likely to find in most market towns is on the car tyres. You'll see perhaps an Indian takeaway, a fish 'n' chip shop and a pub that does sandwiches or a bit of roast beef on Sundays to feed the rural munchers. But before you get too smug about being a townie, there's one type of eating that beats a city gastro-pub in any chompetition: by the seaside.

In general, folk in the country are quite snobby about eating out (that's because the best stuff is cooked at home, the ingredients milked from the local cows or pulled from their own soil. At worst, they'll buy from the farmers' markets nearby). But even if countrymen call 'gourmet pubs' overpriced nonsense, they will drive out of their way to nosh down on scallops, prawns and mackerel by the coast. Having only a few feet to travel from hook to plate, the fish is so fresh you can dance with it.

You can tell seaside eateries that mainly deal with farmers and fishermen as they tend to be stripped down, scruff-as-you-are places – check out The Shed in Porthgain, Wales (a rustic bistro right on the seafront, where the husband catches the fish for the wife to cook), and Hive Beach Cafe of Burton Bradstock, Dorset (staggeringly beautiful beach here, too). If you don't eat anything else here, have the cod and chips and eat it outside with the wind whipping around you. Nothing beats it.

Not that eating by the sea is lacking in style if you want to find it. The East Beach Cafe in Littlehampton, Sussex was designed by architects (Heatherwick Studio) and serves hearty fishy food, with a fantastic view of the sea from all tables. If you do want to dress up (which in the country means holding up your trousers with a belt, rather than string), then go to the Victoria in Holkham, Norfolk – a boutique hotel and a favourite of London's Notting Hill-billies on their bucket-and-spade trip to eat local stylish seafood. Try their pan-fried sea bass with seared scallops. Rick Stein's famous restaurant on the quay in Padstow, Cornwall, has an idyllic setting too. But be warned – it's best to aim for a lunchtime table, unless you've booked months ahead.

Most seaside restaurants do their best to serve only from sustainable stocks, and you may find there's little cod, haddock or plaice on the menu. But plenty of salmon, sea bass, scallops, mackerel, squid, crab, oysters, hake, mussels... Go with the tide: menus change daily, depending on what the fishermen brought in. But don't send the tip in a bottle.

DO

Eat the fish 'n'chips outside – the colder and windier, the better.

Go to Holkham in Norfolk if you're missing your friends in Notting Hill.

Offer to treat your country hosts at a seaside café – it's one of the few rural eateries they won't be sniffy about.

DON'T

Ask whether the lobster screamed as it went in the boiling water – it just upsets everyone.

AUTUMN

25

Taking a Walk on the Wild Side

Walking in the Country

Come September, when the weather cools but the countryside is still lush and beautiful, and especially as the leaves begin to turn golden, even a townie's thoughts turn to long country walks. If you're starting to limber up, you need to plan the outing carefully: a stroll through the paths of our rural lands is not the same as a jaunt through a city park. First off, it's muddy. Forget your high-tech trainers: they might protect you from a tarmac pounding, but they're as much use as an ice-cube in hot chocolate when it comes to walking through puddles. Boots are what you need (see chapter 51).

Once you've got the foot gear and you're wrapped up warm, you can set off. There are rules for walking in the country. Check you are not walking on private land. There are plenty of public rights of way but you won't be the only moving things on them. Footpaths will have other people's dogs running up and down, bridlepaths will have horses (hopefully with a rider still attached) and byways can suffer the earth-churning of off-road cars. With all this action going on, you might be tempted to strike off into a field. Watch out – especially those of you with irritating yippy dogs at your side. The cows don't like them. A townie friend of mine who had taken her noisy terrier along with her for a weekend with friends in Devon was surprised to be asked by her hosts if she was 'all right with cows'. She soon discovered why: as if controlled by a remote switch, a herd of cows turned round as one, loudly mooed and began thundering across the field. She jumped the fence in the style of a matador in a bullring and her dog went missing for three hours.

Country walkers look nothing like ramblers. No socks rolled up over the top of laced-up boots, no matching anoraks, no woolly hats and absolutely no packed sandwiches. Despite the image of hale and hearty countrymen and women, they hardly ever go for a walk just for the fun of it. The only reason they go out at all is to shoot pigeons, or check the fences, or, if it is not a part of their working day anyway, to exercise the dogs. If for some reason they decide they want a spot of exercise themselves, most people I know in the country are happy with a walk around the garden (albeit that most of their gardens are several acres in size). They are also content to do the same walk every day – less boring than it sounds as the joy of the country is that, with the changing seasons, the walk never looks the same twice.

If you walk on the road, be sure to walk on the right-hand side so that cars coming towards you can immediately see you. To be extra safe, when you hear a car, stop and nudge yourself up on to the grassy edge and if the car slows down, stick your hand up briefly to say thank you. If the car fails to crawl past, yell 'Slow down!' and flap your hand up and down to motion them to drop their speed. Of course, they won't take a blind bit of notice but you'll feel much better for it.

Yokels know all their walks and if they're walking on their private land, rarely have to worry about getting lost. But if you are planning to walk for an hour or more, I thoroughly recommend that you take a guide or an Ordnance Survey map with you. Mobile signals are still weak in most off-road areas, and if it's cold at night, you won't want to camp out in an increasingly wet field. Some counties (Sussex, Hampshire, Kent and the Cotswolds – Gloucestershire in case you didn't know – among others) tend to have well-marked footpaths, but most do not.

Keep your eyes and ears open: the odd sighting of a red robin puffing his chest out; the golden corn in the fields just before harvest; the Canada geese flying overhead; a colony of bright green parakeets; even some russet-red rare breed cows lazing in the grass. It's a good reminder that there's more to our world than traffic jams and CCTV.

Finally, remember that even if it's pelting down, a countryman would never open up an umbrella. Just bend your head down and take the punishment – or wear a hoody, if your kids will let you. Always shut the gate behind you and don't drop litter. (Conscientious countrymen never go for a walk without a plastic bag in their pocket so they can collect any they see – and then show it off to their neighbours later. No, not really.) Take my advice: breathe deep and enjoy the clean air. You'll be back in the smog again soon enough.

DO

Wear wellies and wrap up warm.

Take a map with you, if you're not sure of the way.

Keep your eyes and ears open for some amateur twitching (bird-watching, not facial tics). Walk on the right-hand side of the road.

DON'T

Wear a bright-red cape if there are bulls about.

26

Time Travel

Heritage Open Days

It's all very well me telling you to go and play at being in the country for a day or two, but as long as there are gold ropes, watchful guards and tickets to queue for and buy you're never going to feel like a true yokel or rural toff, are you?

Thanks to the joint forces of The Civic Trust and English Heritage (them what protect all the buildings and historical bits and pieces) there is an annual weekend, which is all about heritage for free. To put it nicely, you can go to places that normally aren't open to the public, or where they usually charge for entry, for absolutely nothing. Zip. Nada. Zero. Fancy a country house, a tithe barn or a Buddhist temple? They're yours, my son.

An average 3,500 properties are opened up, with an army of 30,000 volunteers helping to usher the million or so people expected to visit. But it's not just about taking a peek behind the lavishly embroidered curtains. If you go to Broadstairs in Kent, the whole village participates in a two-hour performance in and around the streets, re-enacting the history of their village life. In Sandwich, also in Kent, you can wander around former almshouse cottages (don't pinch the silver). Dorking near Guildford has bell-ringing, a pump gallery and World War II ambulances on display. There are Buddhist temples in the Midlands and the chance to relive your chalky schooldays in an old grammar school at Middleton, Manchester.

These events aren't just for townies: country people go too – who could resist nosying around their neighbours? In fact, those country inhabitants are normally far too snobby to buy a ticket to go round the local stately: they don't want to admit they haven't been invited to step behind the door marked 'private' as a guest. Nor do they want to bump into the lord of the manor while standing on the wrong side of the gold rope (see chapter 4). But with the hordes descending and no money changing hands, they're right there. They might even try looking like townies, so as not to give the game away. If you see someone in a dodgy tracksuit with ten gold chains round their neck and a baseball cap on backwards (that's what they think we all look like), that'll be the farmer from next door. Ah, I jest, of course. But it's worth remembering, sometimes, just what it is that we're all fighting for – go and take a look at our past, present and future.

DO

Lend your countrymen some townie gear – they want the disguise so they can have a gander at their neighbours' houses.

Get a bit het up – for all our modern advances, it's good to know where we all came from.

DON'T

Pinch the silver.

Try to join in the re-enactments if you haven't got a costume on – that ancient blunderbuss will be pointed straight at you and it might still work.

27

All Guns Blazing

Clay Pigeon Shoots

From November until the end of January, if you go to the countryside you'll hear more gunshots than in Manchester's Moss Side. Blasting away animals, small and large, is what ticks many a bumpkin's box. Shooting, my countrymen tell me, teaches a fellow or filly responsibility, hand-to-eye coordination, respect for the land we live in and, above all, it's a jolly good day out. The sport is, in fact, one of the fastest growing in the country – it brings £2.2 billion to rural areas and just over half a million shotgun licences are now held. Perhaps in our increasingly stressful lives the thought of pulverising small flying objects is something of a blessed relief. But you don't have to kill anything to do it. Clay pigeon shooting gives all the fun of the bang with none of the bad karma and, once you get good at it, it is tremendously satisfying.

There are shooting schools all over the UK, often not far from a city centre, yet with views of green and pleasant lands stretching for miles. At the Royal Berkshire

Shooting School, an hour from London, you can turn up on a Saturday and have a proper fry-up cooked by their own kitchens, shoot for two hours and then go and have a gargantuan lunch nearby before driving back to town. Girls shoot too, you know (I think their outfits look particularly natty) and it's probably the best cure for 'bingo-wing' arms I can think of. Boy or girl, if you sign up for a course, it won't be long before you can stand in line without too much embarrassment.

Clay shoots have recently been taken up by the corporate world as a form of posh entertainment and are not restricted to happening in the winter months. Summer shoots are being held more and more, with man-made bunkers to hunker down behind, and clays being let off at random times to imitate the flight of the grouse (which is shot in August), rather than the pheasant. In fact, summer shooting is positively recommended, when it comes to clays, as even very good shots need a few lessons to brush up, before tackling the live birds again.

However, just because the technology is twenty-first century doesn't mean the rules are. Partly because of the dangers of the sport, there are very strict guidelines for shoot etiquette. Between pegs, always carry your gun 'broken' over your forearm, and never point your gun at anyone, even if you are sure it is empty. Clay shoots have also taken on some of the more subtle etiquette of pheasant shoots (see chapter 31). I imagine the rules are shared partly to create an idea of seamlessness between the two types of shoots. At the same time, it is almost inevitable that pheasant (and grouse, woodcock, duck, etc.) shooting will go the way of fox hunting. So there may as well be another ruse to keep the traditions alive, eh?

No need to show up in camo-gear – jeans or corduroys, wellies and a waterproof jacket will do. On a warm day you can wear just a shirt on top, but the guns do press into your shoulders when they go off, so you will appreciate a bit of padding in that area – a waistcoat will do fine. When you hear the instructor shout 'Pull!' it's not a command to snog the nearest person but to announce that the target has just been pinged into the air, with the speed and direction set to mimic a real bird. If you miss, don't worry: you're in line for the Clay Pigeon Conservation Award. That's a little country joke. Ha ha.

DO

Keep up with lessons – even excellent shots need to brush up in the long months between seasons.

Watch out for the force of the gun when you pull the trigger – bruises in the shoulder are common.

Take up shooting if you suffer from 'bingo-wings' – it's the best cure there is.

DON'T

Make eyes at the person standing next to you when the loader shouts 'Pull!'.

28

The Joy of Ceps

Mushroom Foraging

I'm going to put myself out on a limb here and bet that if you've ever walked past a down-and-out rummaging for food in a bin, you've determined that you would never be reduced to such a state yourself. Well, that's as maybe for a townie, but in the countryside people do it all the time. Not rummaging in bins, exactly, but foraging for a bit of free food. If you go down to the woods in the autumn, you won't see bears but men and women crawling in the undergrowth, small bags in one hand, a little knife in the other, scouting for mushrooms.

The ideal conditions for mycologists are a warm September, followed by a golden October. But cep-loving can happen in most autumns, barring extreme weather. Before you go rushing off to find the essential ingredient for mushroom soup, a few fungal pointers.

Where to forage? Forget the alley behind Pret-à-Manger and head for woodlands. Mushrooms flourish in dark undergrowth, beneath beech trees particularly, but a mixed wood is just as good. It's hard to name any precise sites, partly for reasons of conservation (in some places you are forbidden from picking more than 1.5 kg in a day), partly because those otherwise harmless pickers are a fiercely territorial lot. If you spot a Bay Bolete (chestnut-brown cap and stalk, delicious, grows from late summer until first frost, as do all mushrooms), keep it quiet – where there's a single cep, there's bound to be a crop nearby. Don't shout 'Hurrah!' and start pointing, but bend down silently, as if to tie your shoelaces, pluck a few and put them in your bag. Discretion is all.

Before going on a foraging foray, you must learn to identify mushrooms. This is extremely important: it is no exaggeration to say it is a matter of life and death. According to one book of mycology, pick the wrong mushroom for your risotto and there could be 'an onset of vomiting, diarrhoea, sweating and insatiable thirst, followed by a pale, haggard appearance with cold hands and feet, accompanied by a deep state of anxiety. Death can take up to eight or twelve days. There may be a period when the patient feels better. Do not be fooled by this...' and so on. Ruthless dictators could save themselves a lot of money on bombs and just serve up Destroying Angel soup.

Distinctive fungi such as Death Cap (white head and stalk, so named for good reason) and Fly Agaric (looks like a fairy's house with red cap and white stalk, can be hallucinogenic but might be deadly) might be relatively easily avoided but field mushrooms (wide pale caps and pale stalks) could be edible. Or not. It's next to impossible to tell if you're not an expert. The number one safety rule is to NEVER, NEVER, NEVER, pick a mushroom with gills, and don't eat any wild mushrooms raw. This is the recommendation of expert Alexander Schwab who says that this is the only way to absolutely ensure that you never suffer anything worse than mild stomach ache.

DO

Take your first few foraging forays with a guided group before venturing out alone.

Wait until you get home and can cook the mushrooms before eating them.

Take a small knife and plastic bag to conceal your ceps in.

Remember that even poisonous fungi have their uses, as an important part of the life cycle of any number of insects or other creatures, so leave them well alone.

DON'T

Jump up and down with excitement when you spot a cep – you'll get jumped on by your fellow foragers.

29

Bobbing for Apples

Fruit Picking

Within the M25, I don't think you'll find many people who champion the countryside quite as enthusiastically as me. Still, I'm a townie down to my monoxide-poisoned veins and sometimes I find country folk just a little weird. One weekend, on a casual stroll in Suffolk, I came across what appeared to be a motorbike racing driver, complete with trophy, resting on the banks of the road. Further along was Farmer John, astride a child's toy tractor. Just around the corner was Doctor Who and his Dalek, propped up against the village signpost. All of them, and there were 17 more to discover, had straw poking out of every crevice. Yes, this little village was celebrating harvest time with a scarecrow festival and everyone came out to play.

Fortunately, if you want to enjoy the fruits of countrymen's labours, you don't need to ransack your grandad's wardrobe and steal straw: you can just go a'gathering. Those who live out in the sticks relish the month when the air gets crisper and the mornings are colder – the harvest is in, so they can relax for a bit; the countryside looks beautiful (the leaves are beginning to turn golden and there are pocketfuls of conkers to collect) and there is an abundance of food.

Blackberries – best in September – often grow plentifully on the roadside and it's just a question of getting to them before the kids do. Try not to eat too many as you go along – it's embarrassing being spotted by the neighbours with Ribena stains around your mouth, particularly once past the age of six.

Apples are the easiest crop for the common or garden harvester. In fact, there are so many of them I don't even have to pick them. I just walk down the road to my neighbour's house, Bramley Cottage. Every autumn, they put up a sign at the garden gate saying 'Free windfall apples – help yourself' (they even provide plastic bags, bless 'em). Apples get the yokels pretty excited – there's a whole day devoted to the 3,000 British varieties each year in late October. Enough to keep a whole hospital away, let alone the doctor. If you want to make a sweet cider with your apples, this is the best time to pick them too. If you're content just to look at them, and then buy them already picked, go to the very pretty Brogdale orchards in Kent, where they do guided tours through their vast fruit-growing collections – pears, quinces and greengages, as well as crunchy apples.

The easiest way for a townie to harvest is to make like Ma and Pop Larkin and go to a pick-your-own farm. Many close from late autumn until the spring, but some (such as Birchin Lee Nurseries in Sheffield, and JFB Ivens in Peterborough) have fruit and veg ripe for the picking all year round.

If you'd rather grow than pluck, then simply sow your own seeds. That way, you can have your own harvest in your window box or back yard. A fruit tree will take between seven and 10 years to grow.

Later on in the year, those country folk still know how to live off the land. The best way to stave off hunger is to get absolutely blind drunk, so if the harvest has been poor, you only need to attack the sloe gin.

A late, slow autumn is best for an abundance of sloe berries. This purplish blue fruit (or are they seeds? I don't know – I'm a townie, I keep telling you) found on the blackthorn bushes are usually ready to pick in October, but you can still find them well into November, with luck.

Wearing gloves, pick several handfuls and take them home. Folklore has it that you shouldn't pick them until after the first frost, but here's a countryman's tip: just put them in the freezer overnight. This has the same effect, which is to split the skins. Put a couple of handfuls of split sloes into a glass jar or bottle, and cover them with demerara sugar, adding a clove or two if you fancy, maybe some almonds and a stick of cinnamon. Cover it all with gin, filling the bottle three-quarters full. Screw the lid on. Stir (or shake) once every three months. The longer you leave it, the more flavoursome it becomes.

My country food expert also tells me that you can collect rose-hips, haws (the dark red berries on the commonly found hawthorn shrub) and crab apples to make into jelly but admits that this is a 'tiresome process'. So let's leave it to the Hugh Fearnley-Whittingstall fan club.

Finally, remember to watch your manners in the country. If the hedgerows and bushes laden with freebie presents look as if they edge private land, then get permission to pick from them first. And don't be greedy – leave some for the birds and your fellow foragers.

DO

Use the fruit you pick – apples for crumble, sloe berries for gin.

Wear gloves (not woollen ones) if picking any berries.

Pick before the first frost – we've got freezers these days.

Leave alone any birds' eggs or nests.

DON'T

Pick all the apples or berries – leave some for fellow foragers: people and birds.

30

Feeling Horny

Deer Rutting

Valentine's Day is the townie's cue to spray on the perfume, flourish the roses and fend off rival suitors, but in the countryside, they're at it all the time. Not the farmers – although they always seem to be looking for a wife – but the animals. The latter half of September is the turn of the deer and if you go for a walk in the woods then you're in for a big surprise. Not teddy bear picnics but plenty of horny behaviour. (Do be quiet at the back and stop sniggering – I mean *antlers*.)

From late September to early November is the aptly named, in more ways than one, rutting season for our native red deer. The rut is a period when the most impressive stag rounds up a group of hinds (female deer) for mating – think of a cluster of WAGs invited behind the VIP rope for the delectation of a premier league footballer. The challenge is that there is generally a limited amount of hinds to go round, and to stay in control the stag has constantly to drive away his rivals. (The equivalent, perhaps of our footballer spraying

Cristal around the room and threatening to duff up anyone stupid enough to chat up his girlfriend.) The way a stag does this, given the limited amount of expensive champagne to hand in the woods, is to constantly roar. David Tomlinson, *Country Life's* wildlife correspondent, says that, as with some of the more brutish of our football heroes, roaring stags sound like 'bellowing bulls – a primeval sound that makes the hair stand up on the back of your neck'. To up the ante, the stag will rush about, roaring warnings to rivals and thrashing the grass with his antlers. Rutting stags also like to wallow in mud, says David, 'which makes them look even more fearsome, though possibly mud is the equivalent of aftershave lotion and excites the hinds'. The stags do this for as long as they can keep it up and, when exhausted, will be challenged by another stag – this is when they 'lock horns' and fight it out for the pleasure of, well, being pleasured by their chosen hinds later on.

Primeval it may be but deer are not self-conscious animals and you can hear and see this mating ritual in almost as many places as there are nightclubs with VIP rooms. If you take a walk, preferably late in the evening or early in the morning, the sounds of the rut coming out of the mist will be exactly the same as if you had been there in the Middle Ages.

If you're stalking deer, you'll go with a gillie – a guide, who will know the land and the deer better than he knows his own wife. Always take his advice and tip him handsomely at the end of the day. You could try to impress him by licking your finger and sticking it in the air to gauge whether you are downwind or upwind of the stag – but I doubt it would work.

Red deer are magnificent animals, weighing up to 190 kg and, for that reason, the rut is best viewed through binoculars at a safe distance. Our other native deer, the fallow deer, or common park deer, grunt rather than roar but you can still enjoy their antics – even second division footballers can provide a little amusement, after all.

DO

Wear dark clothing.

Take binoculars for some Peeping Tom action.

Stay downwind, if you wish to avoid being attacked by a horny stag.

DON'T

Make any sudden moves.

Say loudly that you'd rather be back at the lodge sipping whisky (the gillies won't like this any more than the stag).

Get too close to a rutting deer – unless you fancy being parent to a mutant Bambi.

31

Shoot-'em-Up

Game Bagging

Perhaps you've bought this book because you've been angling for an invitation to stay with friends in the country. And if you get one, it could be marvellous – all cosy suppers by the Aga, piles of crunchy leaves and crisp country walks. But be wary if asked between November and February. Chances are they'll be asking you to shoot for your supper. Or even, shoot your supper. It's the game bagging season and even if you've never done it before, it's well worth going and giving it, well, your best shot.

If you get invited to a shoot and have never shot before, this isn't necessarily a problem, but you must tell your host and ask for a gun to stand beside you. A 'gun' in this context doesn't mean the weapon itself, but any guest at the weekend who is going to take part in the shoot. Second, arrange to borrow a gun (as in, the real bang-bang piece of work), either from your host or a fellow guest. Third, get kitted out. Go to Beretta in St James's or Cordings in Piccadilly (country people always go to town for their clothes). You don't need to spend a fortune, but wear a good country shirt (a Viyella checked one), possibly a tweedy tie, a round-necked woollen jumper, a warm jacket (tweed or a Barbour), corduroy trousers and walking boots or wellies, although the very smart still wear plus fours. There are girl versions of these outfits too (The Really Wild Company does some great stuff), worth wearing even if you're not shooting.

If you're driving to your shoot, you may spot it ahead of the house when you see fields of what look like forgotten crop – tall dried stalks of maize. The pheasants eat the maize (and there may also be buckets of feed about the place to encourage them to stay there) and then the beaters drive them out of there above the guns.

A typical day's shoot will have about six or seven 'drives' – each drive is an area, for example, 'the high hill' or 'the woods'. A good shoot will have lots of drives of different challenges – high and low drives. You'll see numbered 'pegs', one per gun (there are usually eight guns on a shoot, rarely more than twelve, unless it's a corporate shindig). You'll be given your numbered peg – the place where you stand, usually alone, with the gundogs behind you and the 'beaters' in front. Extremely smart shoots, in the Edwardian style, would have one gun and one loader per peg – and perhaps a butler handing out the bullshots (consommé and vodka).

The best place to be, if you don't want to pull the trigger, is with the beaters: hired hands who go into the woods and drive the pheasants out. Most beaters are old men still working the land – farmers, gardeners, pigmen, estate managers and so on – who are paid £20 for the day, with lunch and wine. But they do it largely because they enjoy the companionship of the day, swapping stories with their fellow countrymen and walking in the fresh open air. As well as flushing the pheasants out, they'll count the shot birds and make sure the dogs pick them up. If you sit in the trailers with them (which take the beaters from one drive to another) you'll get all the juicy local gossip.

As soon as the birds start flying overhead, you can start taking aim and shooting at them. Make sure you only aim for birds in your area – it's considered very bad form to hit another gun's bird. If a bird falls, the dogs and 'pickers' will collect them. Don't shout out if you hit a bird – and especially don't shout that you've hit, when you haven't. Only shoot at the pheasants – no shooting at woodcock, or at 'ground game' – i.e. rabbit – unless you've been told you can.

At about 11 a.m. you'll break for a bullshot and a sausage roll. If not bullshot, you might – at least, if you're at a certain shoot in Norfolk – be offered a sloe gin 'straight', or a 'slowgasm' (a fizzy sloe gin).

Don't brag about how many you've shot, or whine about how badly you're doing. It's not a competition: it's fun. If someone says of your shot, as happened once to legendary country cartoonist Bryn Parry, 'it's a bath bird' – don't worry. It's a term to describe the sort of shot you dream about while lying in the bath.

If you're a girl and not shooting, you'll probably just

go for a walk with the other WAGs and join the men for a drive or two. Remember to stand behind the guns and 'ooh' and 'aah' at their hits and misses so they can feel all big and strong.

At the end of the day, the gamekeeper will come round and tell you how many birds were shot – this is the moment to give him a tip (usually about £20). If this was a corporate shoot, you'll have paid to be there, but if not, your host will have spent a considerable amount of money on the weekend: take a decent present (not pheasant).

LINGO:

'Drive' – six or seven of these in one day – the places where the birds get driven out.

'Beaters' – the people who drive the birds out.

'Pickers' – the people and dogs who collect the shot birds.

'Peg' – where you stand.

A 'gun' – a weapon.

A 'gun' – a guest who is shooting.

'Bullshot' – the typical shoot drink – consommé and vodka.

'Birds' – never call them pheasants.

DO

Wear 'ear defenders' against the big bangs – there are a lot of grumpy old men in the country who refused to wear them in their youth and are now very deaf.

Take a brace of pheasant home (a brace is one hen and one cock), prepared to gut and pluck it yourself.

Refuse to shoot if asked on a Sunday – it's an offence.

Take a tie in your pocket, just in case – look to see if the other guns are wearing them.

Switch off your mobile phone – some landowners fine guests per ring.

DON'T

Turn up with boxing gloves ready to take someone out if you've been asked to be a 'beater' – your job is to flush the birds out from the bushes.

32

Desperately Seeking a Log Fire

Country Pubs

Let's take the most common fantasy: we all know it. You wake up on a freezing cold day. The radiators don't seem to heat more than an inch of the surrounding air in your tiny flat and the nearest you are to a log is the pile of last week's papers by the kitchen bin. You want roaring fires, deep glasses of rich red wine and roast lamb just like your mum made it. So you turn to your partner and say, 'Why don't we find a lovely country pub?' You imagine driving for just an hour or so, through leafy, sun-dappled roads, before chancing a left turn and being greeted by a delightful chocolate-box cottage, with plumes of smoke wafting out of the chimney. Inside a jolly landlord greets you, a bottle of claret open on the bar and a foaming pint of bitter at his elbow, as he nods towards the cosy armchairs by the spitting, glowing fire.

The reality: you are screaming at the satnav as you miss yet another junction off the M3, and the only pubs you can see have 'coaches catered for' signs outside.

You have the choice of eating at a Harvester or a pub overrun by spotty teenagers with New York ghetto rap on a loop. The only food served is a soggy egg sandwich or a microwaved lasagne.

Here's the thing. Idyllic pubs *do* exist as more and more chefs have realised that it is in the countryside that the last remnants of our national cuisine of overcooked cabbage are there to be cleared away – Marco Pierre White, Gordon Ramsay and Heston Blumenthal have country establishments of the inn variety. But these rustic gourmet spots are still relatively rare. You need to rely on a little planning and word of mouth recommendation. Blindly heading for the hills will get you precisely nowhere (or perhaps all roads lead to Harvester).

There are some pubs to avoid, of course. The very remote establishments may not be hugely welcoming to strangers. Most are not quite as bad as those in *Withnail and I*, and as long as you don't walk in wearing a leather gimp suit, you will avoid being stared at. That notwithstanding, I have noticed that strangers won't be served lunch outside the chalked-up hours. The kitchen will close at precisely one minute past three o'clock, and you will be shown a small wicker basket of cheese and onion crisps on the bar, however much you plead that you've been on a long journey and the nearest open shop is 40 minutes' drive away.

This has happened to me. But the best illustration of this concerns the late multi-millionaire Kerry Packer. On a drive back to London from Sussex, with his family in the car, Kerry stopped off at a pub and went in to ask if they could fill up a flask with coffee and make some packed sandwiches for the journey. The landlord said: 'Sorry. The kitchen is closed.' An aide of Kerry's whispered to him that if he could fulfil the order, he would be sure to be handsomely rewarded – this was, after all, the famous and famously generous, Australian multi-millionaire. 'Sorry, sir. You don't understand. The kitchen is SHUT.' So Kerry and his aide walked up the road and into another pub, where they made the same request. 'Of course I can,' said the neighbouring landlord, whose kitchen was also surely shut. 'Hold on, mate,' said Kerry. 'I'll take the coffee and the sandwiches on one condition.' He then slammed several thousand pounds in cash on the bar. 'Go down the road and tell your friend in the pub next door how much I paid you for them.'

DO

Plan your trip – use a guidebook or ask around for recommendations.

Take your dog.

Check the lunch hours before you set off.

DON'T

Expect to pay several thousand pounds for coffee and sandwiches unless you are an eccentric Oz billionaire.

33

Flaming Laughs and Fright Nights

Guy Fawkes' Night and Halloween

I've said it before and I'll say it again: there are some things that only the country is good for. You might not be able to buy a skinny frappuccino or hail a taxi out in the sticks, but you can guarantee pitch-black nights and a cold wintry air. Come the night, cometh the witching hour. And what better place could there be to unleash your screams than in the countryside? All those owls flying about making spooky noises and dusty attics with Miss Havishams walking on the creaky floorboards.

Drive down to the depths of the countryside in the twilight, and you'll find it creepier than fairground ghost trains, with overhanging branches and unknown shadows at the side of the road. My neighbours delight in scaring senseless anyone walking home at night after last orders, with menacing creatures glowing in the window – and the Halloween pumpkins aren't much friendlier.

When you reach the rural hinterlands, you'll find

stately homes all over the country are hosting fright nights and ghostly tours, quite often with a half-bottle of wine thrown in – nothing these country folk like more than a glass to toast to their ghouls. Or you can indulge in a bit of *Blair Witch Project* scariness, with a night walk through the woods. Or perhaps you fancy tracking down bats, armed with just a torch. Got shivers down your spine yet?

Maybe they're braver, or maybe they're nastier, but it seems to me there's nothing a countryman loves more than storing up ghost stories to frighten you out of your wits. As a small child sitting on my grandfather's knee I was regularly petrified by tales of women walking four feet above the floor, children born 183 years ago crying in the night, hanged men appearing at the window... I *loved* it. It's thrillingly easy to unnerve your nerves. Just remember – don't pick up any hitchhikers on that dark drive back.

That pitch-black night is also an essential ingredient for a proper Bonfire Night just a few days later. The best, at least the most exuberant, of these happens in Ottery St Mary near Exeter: a pagan tradition that possibly predates the Catholic-bashing celebration of Guy Fawkes' Night. Whether in a bid to stave off the cold, or just as an alternative to the egg-and-spoon race, the wacky inhabitants of Ottery have been passing burning barrels of tar to each other since the seventeenth century. The ritual involves 17 barrels – each one sponsored by a pub – graded in weight with light ones for women and children (no, I'm not making this up) going up to 30 kilos for the big, strong men. Thousands of revellers line the streets and everyone finishes up at the River Otter with a stupendous bonfire on one side and a funfair on the other. Those crazy kids.

A little closer to the M25 but still more far out than your old man's velvet flares is the gathering in Lewes, Sussex. Thirty-one different societies form individual processions throughout the town, each one with its own rather distinctive look – from Zulus to Vikings, cowboys and smugglers. Six different councils plan for this all year and bonfire enthusiasts start making faggots in August. (Oh, do be quiet at the back – faggots are dry twigs and branches tied together.) Following the true tradition of burning the hate figure of the day as the 'Guy', they like to finish off with an effigy of, say, Tony Blair, Bin Laden or George W. Bush.

If just a normal fireworks night is what lights your Catherine wheel, then there's plenty of those going on around the countryside too (see Directory). It's worth taking the train out of town because the best thing is those dark skies, unpolluted by street lights, which mean you can really see the brilliance of the displays. Bonfires are built by the whole community and, if you want to pitch in, show a little country knowledge by chucking in ash tree branches – the only wood that will burn while still green (handy when there's been a slow autumn a' coming). Finally – remember to burn wood, not animals (those cute furry things that tend to snuggle in at the bottom of the glowing pile). Rocket on.

DO

Check for hibernating hedgehogs before you light the pyre.

Look up into the night sky, relatively unpolluted by electric lights – the best backdrop for stars and rockets.

Help the villagers with their faggots in the weeks leading up to Bonfire Night (note – this doesn't involve either meatballs or public loos).

DON'T

Set fireworks off from a remote Scottish or Cornish island – coastal rescue teams will think it's a distress signal.

WINTER

34

On the Bit

Jumps Season at the Races

The jumps season (flat racing with jumps, not to be confused with point-to-points, see chapter 36) continues all year round, but traditionally kicks off with the Paddy Power Gold Cup, a race at the Open Meeting at Cheltenham, which is held in mid-November. This, according to my jockey-watching friends, is when the racing world really gets excited. They keep up this momentum until the Betfred Gold Cup at Sandown Park at the end of April. Jumps are scarier than flat racing – the races are at least two miles long, sometimes four, and have 'chasers' (big jumps) and 'hurdles' (collapsible fences). Jockeys fall off their horses pretty much as part of the job, but while flat racing is faster, they are much more likely to fall off during a jump, which is more dangerous for both rider and horse, causing a collective gasp amongst the race-goers.

To really get in the swing of things, you want to be in the stands jumping up and down, waving your betting slip and shouting, 'Go, Calypso King!' or whatever the name is that reminds you of your dead aunt's favourite pet, and must therefore be lucky. The easiest way to bet is at one of the lime-green and red tote booths that dot every racecourse. This is the industry bookmaker and the profits are ploughed back into the sport – so if you lose, at least your money is supporting the fun. The minimum bet is £2 'to win' (i.e. to come first), or 'to place' (to come first, second or third) or 'each way' (you hope to come first or second).

You don't need binoculars, just pick out your nag's colours and try and follow them round – the race is over in a flash but the low thud of the gallop as they come round the bend towards the stand is more heart-thumpingly tense than the music to *Jaws*. Listen out for one of two phrases from the crackling tannoy. If the commentator says your horse is 'on the bit', this is a good thing: it means that the horse is going well. If, however, your horse is 'off the bridle', it's going badly, the jockey is shaking the reins to try and push the horse on, as it's getting tired.

The dress code at meets is much less formal than those big summer races such as Royal Ascot, but on the important race days, you'll see a lot of tweed suits. Dress for the elements – no heels on those muddy grasses, and a trilby hat to keep you warm. Tally-ho!

DO

Start to plan how you'll spend your winnings if the commentator says your horse is 'on the bit'.

Bet on the horse whose name reminds you of your favourite pet, rather than waste time studying the form.

Go to the Paddy Power Gold Cup in Cheltenham, which kicks the season off, if you only go to one meet at all.

DON'T

Wear your Royal Ascot outfit to Cheltenham: the Queen is only watching it on the telly.

35

They Shoot Foxes, Don't They?

Hunting

If you live in Britain, you're certain to have an opinion on hunting with hounds. Either you see it as a day out for red-jacketed toffs on horses, bugling their horns, driving protestors into the mud and killing terrified, wheezing foxes. Or it's a marvellous tradition, for sportsmen with a keen sense of competition and a bloody good way to keep those ginger-haired pests under control (doesn't work on Prince Harry, of course, but it does the job with the foxes).

I remember having my first blazing row about the sport when I was in my teens. Stridently, I had declared to my horse-mad hunting friend – following the views of a handsome boy I wanted to impress – that fox hunting was cruel and should be made illegal. She replied that she couldn't possibly believe what I was saying. After all, she claimed, I was a snob, and could hardly deny that all that dressing up stuff didn't appeal: it was about the pack of friends in all their finery, not about the pack of hounds.

The argument, I would say, remains the same even on the national scale. When the hunting ban finally came into force, in February 2005, the question asked was: could the issue of the hunting ban be a cover for a minor class war? It was difficult to believe that the many red faces on the Labour benches of the House of Commons could really be puffed up about a tiny sport that hardly anyone, relatively speaking, participated in. Any countryman I spoke to at the time thought the idea that the Labour government would want to ban hunting on the grounds of cruelty to foxes was so preposterous they wouldn't possibly do it. Besides, whenever the government was under pressure (at the time the ban was imminent, for going to war in Iraq), they rolled out the hunting ban proposal to distract the public from the real issues of the day. If the government needed to bury bad news, they rolled out another dreadlocked hunt protestor and a backbencher MP, who wanted to get his mug on the telly, to call for a new law to stop hunting with hounds. The shock, when the bill finally went through, reverberated through the hills and valleys.

Since the Act of Parliament has been passed, it is apparent that it has failed on every level. Hunting, a sport only ever enjoyed by a minority (about 200,000 people in a population of 59 million), grew its membership by 25% in the three years after the change in the law. As the foxes must now be shot when flushed out, rather than hunted, more are killed during the hunting season than ever before. Only one man, at the time of writing, has been brought to court for flouting the law, and the judge had to throw the case out as it was impossible to clarify exactly how he had contravened the legal position. As for the class issue – that was one that the countrymen passionately rejected from the beginning and are now making moves to make their point visually. The red jackets – correctly called 'pink totes' – are rarely *de rigueur* these days, as hunt members set about de-poshing themselves to encourage as many new people to join as possible.

If you do go hunting (though if you don't know how to ride *very* well I recommend that you only go as a follower, whether on foot or by car), you will be stripped of any notion of hunting as the toffs' sport immediately. Yes, the nobs are there, but so are their staff, the gamekeepers, gardeners and grooms. Not to mention a large number of local riding enthusiasts. The huntsman – who looks after and hunts the hounds – lives on a fairly meagre wage and may come from a farming family, not a landed one. Hunt balls, held now throughout the hunting season to raise money for the hunt, are not full of Ruperts and Arabellas, as Jilly Cooper portrayed, but are populated by every social stratum that the village incorporates. In fact, because the fund-raising entertainment strives to be as inclusive as possible, there are a great many different events, all year – from ferret-racing to formal dinners. If you are new to the country and want to make friends quickly, you can do no better than join the hunt.

But, some will say, what about the practice of blooding? Surely this vile ritual – in which someone who has completed their first successful hunt, smears the fox's blood across their face – marks them out as cold-blooded killers? Well, perhaps there would be a point in this argument. It's a pretty disgusting image. I am assured that this no longer goes on – however, whether this is because hounds are no longer allowed to kill foxes, or whether our twenty-first century mores are being adhered to, is not quite clear.

If you want to go hunting (note – if you would like to make a big *faux pas*, say you are going 'to go to a hunt'), find your local pack from a website (see Directory) and call the Hunt Secretary to find out where the meet is and what to pay. A day's 'cap' will be about £150 for a fashionable pack, and about £10 if you're in Wales. If you want to sign up as a fully-fledged member, an annual subscription will range from £100 to £4,000, although about £1,200 is probably average. It's not cheap, but it's about the same as a season ticket to your local F.C. and you get a lot fitter. Plus, meets are not just on Saturdays – in the peak of the season, you could go hunting three times a week but never on a Sunday.

The dogs employed to hunt foxes (or not, as the case is now) are foxhounds but are only ever referred to as hounds – they are never, *never* called 'dogs' except by hunt saboteurs or ignoramuses. A pair of hounds is named a 'couple' and this is used in the singular: 'Four couple went over the hill'.

So, you're all dressed up with somewhere to go. What to expect? If you have a horse, you'll be up early to get him ready and the meet will be at 11 a.m., either in the village square or at the host farm, or even in the drive of the Big House. If you're staying in the house that is holding the meet, you'll be up early, as everyone stamps about getting terribly excited and stuffing down large breakfasts. The important person is the MFH – Master of the Hounds. If you don't know who that is, ask someone to point him or her out and make a point of riding up and saying 'good morning'. It's a dying practice, but if you do it will mark you out as a townie who knows what's what, as well as someone who has beautiful manners. As a point of etiquette, everyone who hunts does so as a guest of the Master, and the Master is the guest of the landowner.

Young and old trot off – you might see an octogenarian riding out alongside her four-year-old great-grandson – and soon will be galloping and jumping cross-country. For riders, the joy of hunting is the privilege of riding over other people's land at great speed and with several challenges, over hedges, ditches and rolling hills. Landowners will only give permission for the riders to do this in the context of a hunt, making it a rare pleasure. But one hunter told me that the real beauty is in the art of hunting: the skill of responding to the hounds as they follow the trail (now prepared earlier by dragging a smelly rag cross-country). Even if you are not especially genned up on venery (the art of hunting), it is an adrenaline-kicking moment when the hounds suddenly pick up on a scent and make a terrible noise. Few riders who get the hunting bug ever lose it.

Followers enjoy the thrill of the chase by following by car or on foot – although, be warned, if you don't know your way around that part of the countryside, you can get horribly lost very quickly. As with most things, best to latch on to 'Someone Who Knows'. If you are on foot, prepare to feel like a shrunken Alice in Wonderland – for most of the day, everybody will be 10hh taller than you. If you do ride (or follow) across a farmer's land, it is polite to know whose land it is – although the Hunt Secretary will have already secured permission.

If you ride and want to join a local hunt, you are sure to find that you are very welcome. Hunts always welcome new blood and not just of the fox variety (although if you are a foxy type, you are sure to have an even better time). Hunts are wary of saboteurs turning up, so you may get asked a few questions to establish your credentials – don't be put off by this.

But once you're in, I am assured, you couldn't find a quicker way of making friends. Even if you go to another hunting 'country' (in fact, just another pack's area), you will immediately find a friendly network waiting for you. I imagine that the ban has only brought them all closer, in a sort of Blitz spirit.

Those who are very keen to hunt will have a wonderful time. But beware – it is a cliquey society and your status in the hunt will depend on your passion and enthusiasm for it. If you can't talk about hunting all the day long, you could find it very dull indeed. If you fancy the Master, then you really need to be sure you know your foxtrot from your tote – and that's way before you even get to the ball. If you only go once, find a Boxing Day meet. These are the most popular meets of the year, with huge numbers turning up to follow. The sight of a fashionable hunt is striking – with enormous groomed horses, topped by their well-turned-out riders, and the hounds 'singing' in excitement. But even a more low key hunt symbolises the strong community bond and a reclamation of the land by its inhabitants: a synergy between man and animal that has existed for thousands of years. Whether or not you think hunting is right, its place in the fabric of our country, knitting together all ages, all classes and all boundaries, cannot be denied.

DO

Say 'good morning' to the Master of the Hounds.

Pay your 'cap' to the Hunt Secretary – never try to avoid it.

Join in with the other social activities organised by the hunt – you'll make an instant set of friends.

DON'T

Call the hounds 'dogs' and say you vote Labour.

36

Up to Your Hocks in Mud

Point-to-Points

In the bleak midwinter, advocate that I am, even I will admit that there don't appear to be many compelling reasons to go to the countryside. The birds have gone south, the spring lambs are yet to be sprung and the M40 is covered in roadworks. But in the countryside they always find a way to make hay while the sun don't shine. In January, it's all about point-to-points. No, I don't mean sitting by the fire and playing join the dots – it's horse racing.

Point-to-points are steeplechases for amateur jockeys and horses (if you don't think you know what they are, you do – the Grand National is our most famous steeplechase). More specifically, they are there to raise money for, and support, local hunts. The horses in the race must have hunted at least seven times in the current season and the jockey must be a member of, or subscriber to, the hunt. Point-to-points are a big part of the whole hunt scene: everyone involved gets together for a jolly winter picnic, to bet a quid or two and cheer on their favourite jockey.

Point-to-pointing as a sport attracts crowds of about 700,000 every year. But while some of these are large and organised, with a proper race track, stands and permanent bookies, others may have just four horses in the race, a tote van and a car park on a hill for the spectators. Only in December 2005 did the point-to-point season begin before Christmas in Britain, although in Ireland (where point-to-pointing allegedly first began in the mid-eighteenth century) it has started in October for some time. The season runs at the same time as the hunting season, as part of the job of point-to-pointing is to keep the horses fit. Races are usually a minimum of two and a half miles but can be up to four miles long and there are about five or six races in a day – less when it gets dark early. The first race is generally at 12 noon, although from Easter this moves to 1.30 p.m. or 2 p.m. Each car is charged entry (this is partly how money is raised for the hunts), usually about £15 or £20.

Anyone can pitch up to a point-to-point – although you will probably notice that the event is a very matey affair, with people wandering around from car to car, slapping each other on the back and finding an excuse to raise a toast each time. They like to drink at the point-to-point picnics. 'A lot,' one stalwart told me. To look as if you are part of the scene, wrap up warm in woolly scarves, Barbour jackets and scuffed wellington boots. Drive up in a battered Land Rover, with a 'Leave Hunting Alone' sticker on the back window. Preferably accessorise with a muddy dog. Take thermos flasks – one for hot soup, one for hot toddies. Say 'jolly' a lot.

DO

Place a bet – whether it's with the tote van or permanent bookies – just a quid or two is perfectly acceptable.

Take a picnic and lay it out in the boot of your car, offering paste sandwiches and lukewarm soup to all who pass by.

DON'T

Start up a hunting ban debate – especially if you are pro-ban: you'll be used as a jump in the next race.

Be surprised if the affair is fairly amateurish – the race route might be rougher, but probably also much more exciting than anything you've seen on the telly.

37

We do Like to be Beside the Seaside

Winter Beaches

Sticks of tooth-breaking rock, kiss-me-quick hats and the sting of salty air on your face: there's nothing quite like a cold weekend by the seaside. Before you choke on your pretzels, I haven't contracted mad cow disease: this is advice from a genuine countryman. Anyone who lives by the sea all year round will tell you that winter is the time they really enjoy what's on their doorstep. When it's not so cold that your nose is in danger of frostbite but it's just chilly enough to warrant wrapping yourself up in a big blanket and swigging champagne from the bottle as you watch the sun set on the horizon.

In the summer, the beaches of Brighton, Aldeburgh in Suffolk and Rock in Cornwall are swamped with pink bodies by day, and drunken crowds of teenagers swaying around impromptu bonfires by night. Locals stay well away from the beach, only venturing down if they think they can extort some cash in return for ice-cream or deckchairs. The rest of the year, however, you can join them as they walk their dogs, or pitch small tents from which they fish.

Ah, the fish. Even if you don't normally indulge in a chow-down of prawn and monkfish, you mustn't resist the gourmet delights on offer in the seaside restaurants (see chapter 24). Having jumped almost out of the sea and into the frying pan, even the humble fish 'n' chips tastes hotter and crispier when eaten in the cold air. Without the summer hordes you won't have to wait hours to be served either. In fact, all those things that can be too tiresome to wait for in the month of August are a brief joy: have a go at the amusement arcades on Brighton Pier without having to stand behind three hen parties and a gang of schoolchildren high on candyfloss.

If you prefer to take a picnic, then at last you can find a use for the tartan-patterned thermos flask your Aunt Betty bought for you: fill it with hot soup. Choose pebbly beaches rather than sandy ones at this time of year (as at Brighton or Aldeburgh), as the wind will whip the sand up your nose and into your sandwiches. The only question left to ask is: why do some people drive for hours to the beach only to stay inside their cars as they munch on their cheese-and-ham? Answers on a tacky seaside postcard please.

DO

Take a hot flask of soup, cold bottle of champagne and rug – the perfect accompaniments to watching the sunset as you sit on the beach.

Eat in the cold air the very hottest, freshest fish and chips you can find.

Choose pebbly beaches rather than sandy ones in the windy winter.

DON'T

Stay in the car and eat sandwiches – unless your names are Mildred and Harry.

38

No Room at the Inn

Christmas

The countryside really comes into its own at Christmas time. Visions of frost in the morning, carol singers, midnight Mass, home-grown Christmas trees and hand-reared turkeys ensure that everyone strives for a week of Dickensian festivities.

In the country, generally, but particularly noticeable at Christmas, there are two main species: those who have lived in the country all their lives; and townies who are temporarily there to indulge in a fantasy. Townies are easily spotted in the village because they wear tweed, order misshapen veg from the farm shop and plan to roast Bert the turkey from the neighbouring farm. Country inhabitants wear fleeces and trainers, and shop at the out-of-town 24-hour Asda. I have even seen a Tesco delivery van pull up at my village neighbour's front door.

Still, there is no denying that Christmas in the country is a very pretty and cosy time. In a small village, there will be a band of carol singers who go from house to house in the run up to the festivities. You know if you are the most popular house if they finish up with you last, whereupon you must ply them with mulled wine and mince pies, until they are no longer singing carols but a karaoke version of *A Fairytale in New York* and roll out of your front door sometime after midnight.

Log fires blazing add to the romantic vision. These are only recommended, however, if you have fireplaces with working chimneys. To get your logs you can either ask the Big House nearby if they would give you some, perhaps in exchange for a bottle of wine, or you can order some from the local log merchant. Be aware that if you are new to the village (and especially if you only show up at weekends) you will be given the worst wood the logman has in store – wet, or still green (remember, only ash wood burns when green) – which will spit and crackle if you manage to get it alight at all. Only loyal customers are given the good stuff – dry and well cut, with some kindling thrown in. There's nothing quite like the sigh of happiness you will make when your fire catches first time and you are safe in the knowledge that you are at long last part of the local fabric.

But I'm getting ahead of myself. You need to get the Christmas shopping done first, and if you want to fit in, you have to do it in the country. Yes, there are shops in the country: it is not all green fields and fat cows. In fact, I have always thought of country dwellers as somewhat prolific shoppers: it's a social event as much as anything. (Well, they don't get out much.)

All that chatting over the Post Office counter reaches fever pitch when the festive season rolls around. This is chiefly down to the fairs that spring up in every school car park, town hall and stately home. These are local affairs, manned by housewives who want to run a cottage industry of their own and contribute to the family finances. Of course, the stallholders barely break even on their costs as they cannot resist going to all their friends' stalls and spending their profits on them. 'One must be supportive,' they chirrup as they buy yet another overpriced Indian scarf. The Christmas fairs are good if on your shopping list you have: unusual toys for pets, hand-made jam, plant holders, big photographs of dogs, bedlinen and gloves with multi-coloured fingertips. In one trip, I bought soap that looks like big buttons, flower-patterned scissors, a butcher's apron and matchbox covers. You get the picture. You should also find a temporary cafe selling home-made cakes and sandwiches, and a jolly school orchestra to entertain the big spenders.

If you prefer to go to the bigger shops, head off to some of the more pleasant market towns (such as Faversham in Kent, Hexham in Northumberland or Shrewsbury in Shropshire) that more than live up to their name at this time of year. You will find branches of the major chain stores but, more interestingly, there will be plenty of independent shops, more than you will find on a city high street. Their stock will be cheaper than designer goods, often quirkier, and the shopping experience can almost be pleasurable, as it is quieter and less harried. I like to seek out second-hand book shops, cook shops and old-fashioned hardware shops for genuine dad-type gadgets and gardening tools. Besides all this, you will earn the right to wear the insufferably smug look of someone who has not only bought fabulous presents but supported small businesses at the same time. Call it a little present to yourself.

DO

Befriend the local log merchant unless you want to be left out in the cold.

Abandon the shopping list – you won't find anything anyone has asked for.

Welcome the carol singers with mulled wine and mince pies.

DON'T

Surprise your neighbours by entering their house through the chimney.

39

Paint it Green

Arty Weekends

Townies are more comfortable pounding pavements than striding across muddy fields; happier hunting out the latest trendy restaurant than chasing a rabbit down a hole. But at a certain time of year the plethora of feel-good period dramas set in England's green and pleasant fields brings out the yearning for a little rural sport in even the most hardened townie. If the sight of Dame Judi Dench in a frilly bonnet has this effect on you, then pack your bags and whistle a merry tune. It's time for a weekend in the country.

The leaves may be off the trees but the grass is still green on the other side of the fence. The blissful thing about the countryside in the cooler months is the absolute absence of tourists. This is why, if you want to see the landscapes as they were when they inspired our brilliant writers and artists, you should go then (and just squint a bit when a pylon comes into view).

On a cold January morning I went to Flatford Mill

in East Bergholt, Suffolk, to see the scene of Constable's painting *The Hay Wain*. The mill was owned by his father and the young artist made several sketches of the area around the River Stour; the scenes are easily recognisable nearly 200 years later. The visitor centre was shut and the tea shop wasn't serving any buns, but this meant we only spent £2 on the car park (where the attendant had some information brochures for sale, had we wanted them) and were able to enjoy the setting in peace. The land is protected by the National Trust and is clearly enjoyed by the locals. Plenty of people were out walking their dogs across the muddy footpaths and nobody was taking a single photograph.

Similarly, in the winter months, the cottage in which Thomas Hardy was brought up (Lower Bockhampton in Dorset), receives only a trickle of visitors; you can nestle yourself on the windowsill where the author undoubtedly spent many an hour wistfully looking out of the window, dreaming of his faraway lover.

Make sure you take your Wellington boots if you go to any of these spots in the winter as the paths are well worn and the slightest rain turns them into gloopy shoe traps. Stick to the footpaths as some of these go through farmland, and being chased by a farmer on his tractor is no fun (been there, worn the tyre track). Take cash for parking and any voluntary donations requested for upkeep. Take a good dose of patience too – many of these places are staffed and run by locals who take pride in their mini-museums. This means that while there's a lot of love in the room the information isn't always very slickly presented and some of the objects of interest might appeal only to the most obsessed fan – don't laugh, just enjoy it.

DO

Go in the cooler months to tourist hotspots and avoid being trapped in long queues or the camera lenses of a group of Japanese visitors.

Stick to the footpaths of the designated historic areas.

Filter out all modern eyesores with a strategic squint and imagine you have gone back in time.

DON'T

Laugh at the more amateur museum displays – they will have been put together by proud enthusiasts.

Dress up as Peter Rabbit and terrorise the tourists.

40

Galloping Galanthophiles

Snowdrop Meets

You know the first sign of spring is the cuckoo's call. And you've heard of the first swallow of summer. Hardened townie though you are, even you will know that in autumn the leaves on the trees turn golden. But I'll bet you didn't know that a sign of winter is large crowds of bottoms sticking in the air, heads close to the ground, with just the faint sound of muttering and the occasional 'ooh' or 'aah' to be heard.

These rotund displays can be seen across the countryside in February, gathering in a mob-like fashion. At any moment, large numbers of people – all enslaved by their common passion, which many have likened to a cult – will suddenly collect to peer at snowdrops.

This is a regular homage to that little miracle that happens every winter, when even the most barren ground pushes through delicate posies of delight. These tiny white flowers inspire an 'affliction' known as Galanthophilia, an addiction to the looking at and growing of snowdrops. The, er, medical term (and I'm not making this up – well-known gardeners will happily use the word) comes from the official botanical name for the flower, *Galanthus*. Which, confusingly, actually translates as 'milk flower'.

My galanthophile friends tell me there are 20 known species of snowdrop but more than 500 varieties. Which rather implies that there could be other snowdrop species lurking in the undergrowth, just waiting for that eureka moment of discovery by a passionate plant worshipper. At least, unlike the orchid hunters, there is little chance of getting kidnapped by guerrilla groups in a Cotswold 'jungle'.

Galanthophiles come from all botanical walks of life – from the professional to the amateur, the stately home to the council estate. The cult is referred to by plant boffins as 'democratising'. You may think that any appreciation of nature is 'democratising'. After all, trips to the countryside regularly result in all manner of us over-enthusiastically exclaiming over green grass, blue skies, moo-moo cows and little lambikins. But the problem for a galanthophile is that rich or poor, vast sums of money need to be accrued to buy a prime snowdrop bulb. Just one bulb can cost up to £30. Some do cost just a few pence each from Woolworths, but the best bulbs have taken four years to be ready for sale and will repay you with a glorious display for decades.

Henry Elwes, the great grandson of a famous snowdrop collector (there is a bulb named after him) runs the most beautiful snowdrop garden in England at Colesbourne Park, Gloucestershire, and has been host to the cultish galanthophiles for many years. Up to 1,600 followers can turn up in one afternoon and, while most of the crowds are dispersed, there will be the occasional pinch points over certain exciting hybrids. No shoving allowed. Touching isn't strictly forbidden, but they don't really like it – however, if you're a snowdrop boffin, you probably want to turn up the flower-head and look inside for the markings. It's all about the markings. If you're not a boffin but want to pass yourself off as one, talk about whether the flower-head has green on the inside, or outside, is wholly white or wholly green. You may eventually learn to distinguish between 250 different varieties, as Henry can. You can also talk vaguely about how it is thought that the Romans brought over the first wild snowdrops – although we think of them as quintessentially English, they are in fact a Mediterranean flower. If you want to be completely cast out of the galanthophiles' world, excommunicated if you like, simply pick a couple of the snowdrops and pocket them.

Traditionally, snowdrops flower in February, but in recent years (yet more grist to the mill of global warming) they've begun in mid-January. So if you want to get out to a snowdrop meet, wrap up warm and take your own sandwiches. Don't forget to wear fingerless gloves, so you can touch these legendary flowers with the caution and gentleness they deserve. Much as you might touch the body of the god you worship.

DO

Treat the flowers with loving and gentle care.

Expect to shell out a small fortune if you want to cultivate your own floral winter wonderland.

Refer to the Roman invasion, and how they brought not just straight roads and plumbing but also the *Galanthus*.

DON'T

Pluck any of the snowdrops and pocket them – you'll be outcast faster than you can say 'milk flower'.

Shove your fellow galanthophiles aside so you can peer at the inside markings.

41

Tossers

Pancake Day

If you're going to the country for the weekend, make it a long one and stay there for Shrove Tuesday. All over England's bonny lands rural types will be flipping pancakes in the open air. In Olney, Buckinghamshire, one of the oldest pancake races known to exist has been held since 1445. Apparently it was a very cheering event for the womenfolk left behind during the War of the Roses. Just because they're flipping, doesn't mean they don't flipping care. One year, a three-time winner (running the 415 yards in 63.76 seconds) was banned from entering, to give the other women in the village a chance.

Only women may enter the race: they must be over 18 and have lived in the town of Olney for at least three months. No lycra here either – all racers must wear the traditional costume of the housewife, including a skirt, apron and head covering. (The rules do say, though, that they don't have to be married. People outside the big cities can be liberal thinkers too, you know.) Of course, they must also be flipping a pancake. Winners have not only to cross the finishing line first but also toss their pancakes before being given a kiss by the vicar – called the Kiss of Peace (actually, I think that might be a handshake). But they also get the traditional prize of a kiss from the verger. Ooh-er!

While pancake races have been run through wars and pillaging, it's the twenty-first century's health and safety rules that are causing the tossers to stick their pancakes on the ceiling. Okehampton Primary School's annual race in Devon was threatened by 'spiralling' insurance costs a few years ago. They were also told that 25 marshals would be needed to man the 50-yard course, 'to ensure public safety'. Fortunately, a local pancake lover stepped in at the time to pay the bill and negotiate the number of marshals, and it is now paid for by the local council. I am assured that despite these hurdles, teachers and pupils will pitch up to run and flip pancakes in a daredevil combination of hand–eye–pan coordination, even if it's half-term.

Pancake racing requires skill. This fact the Dean of Worcester Cathedral discovered at the race to launch an appeal for his place of work, when, as the local paper so beautifully put it: 'the Shrove Tuesday sprinter finally fell on the fifth lap in a flailing flurry of fabric'.

Some villages can't wait until Shrove Tuesday itself, and will hold the frying pan based festivities on the weekend before. At Trowbridge, Wiltshire, they promise that their traditional 'pancake racing hasn't changed much … it's still as funny as ever'. There are races for women, men and children, as well as pancake relays and pancake making on the spot. Take care if you go there: nothing stands in the way of a countryman and a day of full-fat celebrations.

DO

Take your own frying pan (and toppings).

Challenge health and safety officials if they're trying to stop tossers from having their fun.

Leave the lycra running gear at home.

DON'T

Eat your pancake until you've run the race.

Slap the vicar when he kisses you – it's the prize for winning the race.

If you're a man, wear drag to enter the Olney pancake race – only a full transsexual operation will fulfil the terms of entry.

PERENNIALS

42

Roses Round the Door

Buying Your Dream Cottage

So you can't go on holiday abroad any more, for fear of the mess your size 16 carbon footprint will leave behind. Holidaying in Britain is the 'green' answer but what if a B&B in Margate that smells of cabbage or a hotel run by Basil Fawlty doesn't float your cruise liner? You need to make like the country folk and have a place of your own there.

Townies have long been able to cash in on their escalating equity and put down a sizeable deposit on their dream cottage (thereby outpricing the yokels). But before anyone starts smelling the roses, you need to get pricked by a few thorns first.

Where to go? There are 'hotspots' in the country but do you want to bump into your fellow Glaswegians or Notting Hill-billies at the local post office? Aldeburgh in Suffolk is known as 'Chelsea-on-Sea', for example. And I've bumped into more friends in Bridport, Dorset, than in Piccadilly Circus. Even the coast of Wales, because of its beautiful surfing beaches, is quietly becoming a hang-out for trendy urbanites from Bristol, London and Manchester, and, therefore, appropriately expensive. (But watch out if you're looking to invest – most Welsh properties are cheap now and will stay that way for many years.)

Next to consider: do you want to be isolated or not? In town your main concern is to be near a station and kebab shop. But in the country you probably think you want to be as far from the main roads and villages as possible. But those tiny roads that separate your house from the noisy main road are often full of holes, guaranteed to destroy your car unless you crawl along at 3 mph. Not to mention that, being so far from the village, you will have to get in a car and drive for 15 minutes, at least three times a day, just to get a pint of milk or newspaper.

Large gardens for games of croquet may be part of your weekend fantasy, but unless this image includes several hours of mowing with a rusty machine, I'd avoid too much lawn. Any gardening at all can be nightmarish, unless you are there all the time or can employ a gardener. I only have two pot plants and some supermarket herbs to manage on a weekend basis and I find that ridiculously stressful. Large areas of land should also be considered carefully. A friend of mine in Wiltshire loved one house she found but was a bit unsure about the occasional dodgy whiff that blew past. The estate agent dismissed it, but an investigation revealed the garden was atop a toxic landfill site. Another thing to check is whether your backyard is part of the Ramblers Association's map of Britain. Madonna suffered this ignominy when she moved into her Wiltshire manor. If your cottage is on the map, you'll need to make sure you've got a dressing-gown on over your birthday suit when you fetch the milk off the back step in the morning to avoid giving any passing walkers a nasty shock. And you may dream of growing your own Sunday lunch but if you want to use your land to keep animals, even a humble hen or two, then check with the local council that you have permission.

Should you find what looks like a charming historic cottage – beware. Some quite cheaply priced dwellings may be Grade II listed, meaning that the tiniest change to the house will require local planning permission, or the nod from a body such as English Heritage. This can be costly and frustrating; one happy couple I know in Dorset have seen their plans crumble over four years of seeking approval.

Arm yourself by befriending local estate agents who will know the lie of the land and its inhabitants well. Or go through a buying agent, who will filter through potential problems for you. Finally, of course, always get a proper survey – ancient plumbing, ambitious wiring and the constant threat of damp and woodlice aren't always visible. Nonetheless, no survey will reveal the 93-year-old one-toothed housekeeper you'll be expected to employ at an extortionate rate, just because she comes with the house. Happy hunting.

DO

Consider employing any staff employed by the previous house owners.

Get a proper survey done.

Think carefully about how much gardening you can manage.

Check whether your prospective rose cottage sanctuary is on a public right of way.

Talk to local pub landlords and villagers to get the lie of the land.

DON'T

Ignore the dodgy whiff in the air – it could be infinitely more toxic than the cows in the field next door.

Live too far away from the village if you have neither car nor bike.

Buy in a trendy part of the country if you're trying to get away from your townie mates.

43

Back and Forth

Commuting

Chances are, if you've bought, rather than inherited, your house in the country, you'll have a massive mortgage. So before you can enjoy an unadulterated 24/7 rural existence, you'll still be commuting to town for work. Commuting is, in fact, a large part of many countrymen's lives. Indeed, they have found a way to incorporate it into their social timetable, using the hours spent waiting on the platform or sitting on the train as an opportunity to catch up or show-off to their peers.

Commuters from the smaller stations will have fewer trains to take them into work, which means that a routine will be quickly established. Leave the house at 7.08 a.m. precisely, drive to the station, park in the same place as always, quick-step to the platform, wait in the usual spot, nod to your fellow passengers and all aboard at 7.46 a.m.

It's harder to find a regular waiting spot at the larger stations, but a frequent commuter will have his own routine once aboard and will recognise most of his co-travellers – only he is less likely to chat to them. I've been elbowed out of the way of a space by the train's bar on the 18.11 train from Liverpool Street to Colchester, by a man who clearly liked to park himself there Monday to Friday with two cans of Stella and the crossword.

On the other side of the tracks, for two years of commuting between Ladbroke Grove and Southwark Tube stations in London, I saw the same woman travelling to work. She must have been a near neighbour, and we certainly worked for the same company – yet in all that time, we have never got further than a tiny nod and smile of recognition. Were we to have been travelling companions between Little Riding and Waterloo, we would almost certainly have struck up a conversation after a few months (or less). Many firm friendships begin on the 8.23.

Delays and engineering works, wrong type of leaves and snow and so forth notwithstanding, on the whole a commuter's life is a regular one and I am told that once you get into the rhythm of it, you can stand quite a long commute; if you are lucky it becomes a part of your day that you barely have to think about. One former colleague of mine commuted from Bournemouth to London, spending over four hours on a train daily. He said he had learned to fall asleep the second he sat down and only wake up at his station. The pay-off, of course, is a bigger house than you could afford in a city centre, and the sheer pleasure of being in the country when you wake up on Saturday morning.

But there are also some interesting subtleties of snobbery on trains. For a start, there's the first class and economy divide – as gaping a chasm as anything suffered by gentry and serfs in medieval times. The first time I took a train journey alone, I had been taken out to a very posh restaurant by my uncle, and was on my way to stay with even posher cousins near Hungerford. When I got the train, I saw the stickers on the windows saying '1' but assumed that was the number of the carriage and sat down. I was the only girl in the carriage and a teenage girl to boot. I remember the older businessmen smiling at me rather quizzically. Well, I thought, I don't really know what all the fuss is about with trains. It was on time and very comfortable; I could even have coffee in a china cup, and there was plenty of room...

Until the conductor came round. Upon which I was immediately thrown into the carriages beyond and found myself squashed between two screaming babies, a granny and a small child playing drums on my knees. *Then* I saw what the fuss was about.

The difference in cost is extortionate between first and second class – but, by golly, if I had to commute every day and I had the money to do it, that's the way I would travel. Nevertheless, while this is true, the comfortable conditions are only part of the reason why commuters pay over the odds. Mostly it's to do with showing off. Well-to-do businessmen in the City like to sit there, safe in the knowledge that they are away from the *hoi polloi*, sitting amongst their peers, indeed probably sitting with friends they had dinner with the night before. Deals can still be done on the 18.36.

But it's not only sitting in first class that marks you out as a success in some eyes. It's the ticket you hold. A friend was holding a business meeting with a colleague on a trip, but was disturbed throughout by the noisome snoring of the only other man seated in the first-class carriage. Shortly after the portly gentleman awoke, my friend's mobile went off, which he answered. Naturally, there was a scene about who had caused the greatest disturbance, which the snorer settled by announcing as he walked out, 'But *I* am a season ticket holder!'

Then, of course, there is the station you get out at. Main commuter stations (Reading, Colchester, Woking) are deemed to be 'a bit minor public school' and the snobs will go out of their way to disembark at somewhere rather more genteel and small, to indicate that they live in an enormous house in the middle of nowhere.

As a small point, I know this applies to any train journey, but talking on mobile phones really *is* irritating. Longer train journeys can mean that travellers feel more relaxed and tend to hold longer conversations. I'm writing this from a train, and on the next table a man is having a full-length chat with a friend, detailing his extensive plans for building works on his house. I couldn't help but smile at the woman opposite when we heard him say, into his hands-free set, with some force, 'But look, don't tell *anyone* about this, yeah?'

The radio DJ Johnny Vaughan, however, has the best advice for train travel. To discourage anyone from sitting next to you simply smile directly at them as you pat the space beside you.

DO

Book a first-class ticket if you want to wear your success on your sleeve.

Establish a routine quickly – same parking spot, same train, same seat.

Chat to your fellow commuters, particularly the ones you work with.

DON'T

Use live weapons to defend your usual parking spot/seat on the train/spot in the buffet car.

44

Wild Rover

Dogs

If you've got a dog in the city, every now and then it's only kind to give it a break and take it out to the country. It's a dog's life in town – not just the hard pavements on your pooch's paws, or mangling its legs on escalators – but for you, picking up its poo and putting it in a plastic bag. It's enough to turn you to taxidermy.

Country people love their dogs and their dogs love them right back. In fact, country folk would rather send their children away (they call them 'boarding schools') than pack their dogs off to kennels when they go on holiday.

But just as the people do things differently in the rolling fields of Britain, so do the dogs. Country dog-lovers like their dogs to be working animals, trained to round up sheep, protect the chickens, chase hares, fetch shot pheasants and ward off intruders. You may think that your precious pet, Snuffles the Shih Tzu, who has dined exclusively on grilled chicken all his dog years, wouldn't notice the presence of a live feathered version, but you would be wrong. Primitive canine instincts may suddenly reveal themselves in a red-blooded mist. If you don't want to spoil lunch with your friends in the country by providing the main course unplucked and in shreds, not to mention ahead of schedule, I recommend that you keep your pawed pal on a leash.

When staying with two-legged friends in their country abode, make sure you've let them know in advance that you'll be bringing Rover with you. Bring your own supply of dog food and water bowl. If your dog has a tendency to chase cats/bite small children/chew shoes then you need to take a travel box for him to stay in, too. (Don't leave dogs in the car, even with the windows open they can get hot and very, very bored.) And remember that while people in the country love their dogs, they are unsentimental about animals: giving your dog scraps from the dinner table will get you both sent to the kennels.

Out in deeper countryside, on public paths, feel free to let the bitch off the leash. (Fill in your own wife/girlfriend joke here.) However, be aware that the wide, open fields (especially between March and August) are not your dog's own personal playground. No farmer will smile indulgently when your poodle has barked at the sheep or worried the cows. In fact, in some cases, a farmer is legally entitled to shoot a dog that is chasing his livestock. One friend of mine was exercising a friend's dogs by having them run beside her car as she drove up a long driveway. Slowly becoming aware she was being watched, she looked around to find armed gamekeepers standing in the woods with menacing glares trained on her noisy mutts. She hastily gathered them back into the car before blood was spilled.

If you want a dog that fits in with the countryside look, you'll need to ask around to see if there are any local breeders. The buying and selling of dogs tends to happen through word of mouth. The most popular country dogs are still Labradors by a long chalk – they work hard, are easy with children and love attention. Lurchers and cocker spaniels are also sought after. Jack Russells are also a prime choice for a country dog owner – great for long walks but the yippy barking can become a little irritating. (This is just a personal opinion, of course, and one, I might add, that I freely apply to all terriers and other bad-tempered little brutes.)

Finally, your dog may be used to sleeping at the end of your bed but in the country they'll be kept in cages at night, or in the stables outside. Don't fret. It's a dog's life, and they're used to it – or soon will be.

DO

Remember to take with you: a leash, bottle of water, dog biscuits, a water bowl and possibly a travel box.

Remember that it is sometimes legal for farmers to shoot to kill any dog that is worrying their livestock.

Talk to a local dealer or rescue home if you want a country dog.

DON'T

Applaud and shout loudly when your dog chases the sheep.

46

The Farmer Wants a Wife

Dating

Townies have a smorgasbord of snogging opportunities available – from dating in the dark to lunchtime hook-ups. But what does the farmer do when in need of a wife? Or even the townie in search of a little country life and love?

Farmers have had a sympathetic ear for some time when it comes to matters of the heart, with various magazines and TV shows launching campaigns to find them a wife. It must be harder for the silage worker, grave digger or post office manager. (Incidentally, what does anyone ever do for dustmen? When people say, 'I'd love him *even* if he were a dustman', do they think about how hard it must be for them to get a date as it is?) Not quite so tricky, of course, you would think, for the posh estate owner; but while he may have an impressive threshold to carry the bride over, she'll never wear a jumper without holes in it again or know a bedroom where the ice doesn't form on the inside of the window. Big old house equals no dosh.

Oddly, given the pace of life for country folk, speed dating is all the rage. There are organisations that set up speed dating events all around the countryside and you can find yourself a hottie from Rutland to York. If you travel up from town, they'll probably be beside themselves to see you. As one lovelorn dater from Shropshire told me, 'The problem is, in a village, the same people come round every time.' Less a speed date than a conveyor belt.

Roger Scruton in *News From Somewhere* writes that ten years or so ago when he first moved to the country, the lonely hearts page in *Farmers Weekly* was full of farmers detailing their vital statistics (acreage, quality of soil), and looking for marriage. Now there is just a small corner of ads offering 'post-modern relationships' and Thai brides. Actually, online dating is a growth industry in the country. Lonely goatherds online do things differently – profile pictures are more likely to be of their horse/dog/sheep than of the lovelorn themselves.

But a good place to find a bumpkin in search of love is the decent bar in any market town – there's only ever one decent bar, so it's not hard to find – on a Tuesday or Thursday night. You'll see plenty of nervous singletons fiddling with their white wines or pints of bitter, as those are the nights they set up their blind dates. Presumably at the weekend they're too busy milking cows to be fondling anything else. You need to be gentle with these rural souls: their singles events are as much about being sociable as landing Mr or Mrs Right Now. Forget the New York job interview style of dating and don't seek to impress with overly complicated cocktail requests or a hip outfit that requires a degree in origami to put on (or take off, for that matter). Instead, ask nicely about their families – all of whom will live in the same village and are probably watching your every move on a webcam – and show off your fetching rubber. Pair of boots, that is. Ooh, you are naughty.

DO

Join in with gusto – if the same people come round every week on the speed dating conveyor belt, ask more inventive questions.

Approach the dating scene lightly – it's as much about making friends as love.

Ask nicely about their families – they're probably watching you from the bar.

Avoid asking every farmer you meet if he's looking for a wife.

Stick to comfy country clothes – townie outfits frighten the horses (and the men).

DON'T

Marry a man for his acres: just like the proverbial six inches, they may yield less seed than you might expect.

46

I'm a Celebrity, Let Me In

Famous and in the Country

You're rich. You're famous. You finally made it. You won *The X Factor*, scored the goal that won the FA Cup, wrote the movie that broke box office records, accepted the BAFTA, managed the England team that brought home a trophy, designed the fastest car or simply married someone who had done one of the above. You've bought the diamonds and the boob job, snorted a small Brazilian mountain, walked down the red carpet and sold your wedding to *OK! Magazine*. What next?

Historically, the rich and successful have always liked to put the seal on their status by buying, or building, a stonking great pile in the country – from fiefdoms conferred to illegitimate sons of kings to the Victorian industrialists and the early stars of screen and stage. After World War II, when the social fabric began to change radically, any snobbish means of showing-off lost favour. Anyone who inherited a manor couldn't afford to run it because of newly legislated crippling death taxes. If you were lucky enough to be able to buy a big house in the country in the 1960s or 1970s, it was probably because you wanted the 'good life', complete with home-grown marrows and your own chickens.

But the increasing rise of the super-rich in the fields of sport and television, as well as the City, has meant that many people have started to look again to the country as another fabulous way to spend their money, while wearing tweed caps and pretending to live the good life too. The fact that their organically grown veg are tended by gardeners, or their stables managed by grooms, is kept quiet. Some celebrities like to buy their piles in order to emulate the lords of the manor of yore – Madonna, Elizabeth Hurley, Sting, Alex James and Kate Moss to name a few. They host shoots on their land, make their own cheese and can be seen drinking ale and wearing wellies, as well as taking the opportunity to praise the 'normal' life and their village friends (a.k.a. 'civilians') when interviewed.

One celeb of my acquaintance says that the important thing is not to be disappointing. While there may not be the time to go to all the events in town, in the country a local celebrity should open the local fête, or hold a Q&A session for the WI. Elizabeth Hurley almost got it right when she switched on the Christmas lights of her local Gloucestershire village; but, unfortunately, she forgot that she couldn't then behave like a 'normal' person by donating kneelers to the church she got married in, instead of the million quid they were expecting.

There are some in the A-list who simply want a grand house – the very biggest they can find, with their newly created coat of arms on the gate, a security system that would outdo Fort Knox and an outdoor swimming pool heated for all 12 months of the year. These landowners tend to be glamour models or footballers and their WAGs (most notably Wayne Rooney and Coleen McLoughlin, and David and Victoria Beckham) and are rarely spotted down the pub.

But for all these celebrities, despite having escaped to the backwaters, they still face the same pestilent problem they have in town: the paparazzi. Snooping journalists will crawl round the village, talking to the pub landlord, the village postmistress and the bobby on the beat, trying to find out the movements of the hot stars. A great big driveway is no hindrance to the long lens. So, if you are rich and famous and you've just moved into the idyll of your choice, you need to get the local villagers onside – *immediately* – so that they will feel more loyal to you than to the colour of money.

To this end, a local celebrity should try to help out local people where possible. A successful scriptwriter I know will generally refuse the long stream of requests to read scripts, cast a friend as extra and so on. But if someone asks who lives in the close vicinity, he says he will do what he can to give them a leg up. Which is nice, don't you think? He says he does it partly so as not to be snotty, but admits that in another sense it could be rather paternalistic (particularly if said celeb lives in the biggest house in the village).

Whether you are a pop star or playwright, be sure

to *use* the village – go to the post office, the local shop, buy the farm eggs and pop into the pub for a pint or pre-walk Bloody Mary now and again. Secondly, employ locally – you might want to bring in a super-trendy interior designer to overhaul your mansion, but you need to use the local painter and decorator to put it all in place. This also goes for tradesmen – builders, plumbers and electricians – particularly if you're doing major works on the house. Remember that *you* are providing the stories that the workers will tell down the pub, when they get asked (as they surely will) 'what is he *really* like?'. Make them cups of tea, buy decent biscuits, ask after their families and give them a really good send-off lunch when the work has been done. On a smaller level, you also need to employ your daily cleaner, gardener and so on from the village. The best way to do this is to find one person you really trust in the area, and get recommendations from them. Pay generously. At Christmas, always tip the dustman, the milkman and the newspaper delivery man.

Finally, befriend some of the villagers. You can either host a great garden party once a year, or even better, get to know a few people that you can invite for Sunday lunch or supper a couple of times a year, when you've got a famous mate or two over at the same time. In other words, you need to treat the villagers much as you would journalists – by using tactics to keep them onside. But eventually, I hope, you will become genuine friends and when the paparazzi come calling, they'll be chased out of the village faster than a raging bull through a gate.

DO

Open the local village fête or switch on the Christmas lights (this is especially useful if you need planning permission from the council for any changes you want to make to your house).

Splash your cash by employing any staff locally.

Remember that you may have moved to the country to be 'normal' – but no one else will see you that way.

DON'T

Turn up to open the new supermarket with bodyguards, hairdressers, publicists and paparazzi in tow.

47

Cooped Up

Keeping Chickens

As a nation, the British are chicken crazy. We eat nearly 26 million eggs a day and the white meat is consumed with alarming frequency – from nuggets to roast. But are we loving the hens? Is the cockerel getting the affection he needs? Judging from the fact that 70% of our eggs are supplied by battery hens, it would seem not. Of course, this is only really an issue for townies. In the country, people don't buy eggs from the local supermarket, they collect them from their own roost. If you want to know where your eggs come from, you can't do better than go looking in your own backyard.

Just like dogs and sexual partners, you need to pick the breed that is right for you, perhaps even looks a little like you. The Ancona hen is beetle-green with mottled feathers but not just a pretty beak, producing up to 160 eggs a year. The Cochin is tall and haughty looking with soft feathers all the way down to her chicken feet, but is so friendly she is likely to be caught by a fox.

Unless you want to breed chickens, no cockerel is necessary (and if you have neighbours, positively discouraged, unless you actually want to disturb them at dawn, of course).

The chicken that comes in a bargain bucket with chips, will probably have been intensively raised and fattened in five or six weeks. But a home-grown hen shouldn't be killed until it's about three months old. They will need a protected enclosure and some space to run about, with a plentiful supply of clean water to drink. You can feed your chickens with tidbits from the dinner table – creating a perfect circle from scrap to chicken to scrap again. They especially like greens, bread soaked in water, plus wholesome chicken feed (maize is best). Once they've grown fat enough and before they start trying to mate (they won't get fatter after they've got their leg over), they're ready for the roasting tin. The brave snap their necks cleanly with their bare hands. The less brave e.g. me – ask someone to do it for them. The foolhardy leave it to the fox.

The fox is a perilous and pestilent enemy of our feathered friends. Chicken wire or a decent coop might keep them out but hens are sociable creatures, who enjoy running about, scratching for food and having the odd dust bath. Keeping them under lock and key is no fun. One Suffolk farmer recommends hanging a portable radio, switched on, in a plastic bag by the coop, tuned to Radio 2 – apparently foxes particularly dislike the sound of Terry Wogan's voice.

DO

Provide your hens with plenty of water and a big bowl for them to have dust baths.

Kill them at the right time and as swiftly as possible.

Name them and remind everyone at lunch just who you're eating – it's the country way.

DON'T

Let them out loose beyond the run if you can't keep an eye on them – the fox will snap them up quicker than you can say 'cluck off!'.

48

Four Fingers Good

Driving on the Open Road

You love driving; you hate traffic. You've spent all your hard-earned cash – or at least, committed to a never-ending series of monthly payments – on a beloved old banger/roaring speedster but, driving in town, you can rarely go faster than 7 mph, which hardly burns the rubber. Quite frankly, your car might as well be a motorised armchair. When the sun is shining, what could be better than a beautiful drive to the country? The open road, the wind in your hair and a sublime absence of speed limits.

Let me just ask you to make an emergency stop there. You see, driving in the countryside is full of tiny little rules that you won't find in even the small print of the *Highway Code*. First off is the Country Law of Overtaking. This is very simple: there isn't any. As soon as you turn off into one of those delightful tree-lined roads, you'll notice that they are hardly wider than a single lane and have more bends than a charmed cobra in a basket. And driving on this road will be Tractor

Man, an extraordinary specimen, who not only phut-phuts along at walking pace, but remains oblivious to the long queue of cars behind him, stretching into the next county.

My fellow countrymen have also pointed out a particular peril of driving in the country: you share the tarmac with any number of things that, in town, would normally be safely shunted on to the pavement: walkers, dogs, cyclists, children. Driving round a corner means you run the high risk of crashing into any one of them (I've nearly careered into horses more than once), not to mention oncoming cars that you can't see. For this reason, I actually prefer driving at night in the country – the headlights mean you can see when a car is coming well before it actually turns the corner.

So, you may as well sit back and enjoy the view. But even here, danger lurks. A survey revealed that one in ten drivers lose their concentration on the road because they are so diverted by the scenery. With 16,000 serious accidents on rural roads each year, perhaps all side windows should be blacked out. At the very least, if you don't want to lose your no-claims bonus you had better stay away from the pretty fields and moo-moos, and drive to that lovely village pub instead (see chapter 32).

But villagers have long been infuriated, if not actually mown down, by cars speeding through their picturesque streets. In retaliation, many have installed large signs that flash 'SLOW DOWN!' in embarrassingly bright neon. They are not speed cameras but are probably more effective.

Once you've slowed down to drive past the villagers, you can now observe the Country Law of Saying Hello. In town, if you see a friend, you wave frantically, toot your horn and shout out toodle-pip or some such jollity. In the country you must do only the following: very, *very* slowly raise four fingers off the steering wheel, accompanied by a *slight* nod of the head. (Bill Bryson has noted that in Yorkshire the wave is just a single finger raised, and this modest greeting is awarded only to those who have been accepted into the local community after several years.) Note that, apart from in Yorkshire, this greeting is standard to everyone: from the person who gave you the price of eggs in the village shop that morning to your dear old mum. When I first started living in the country, I thought that my boyfriend knew an awful lot of people as on our walks he said hello to everyone that walked or drove past – of course, he knew almost no one at all.

It's worth being friendly, by the way, as you'll probably run out of petrol and need rescuing. Rural petrol stations are few and far between – over 200 have closed down in England and Wales since 2000 – and they are not open 24 hours with fully stocked supermarkets and coffee bars attached to them. Of course, you could just take the train.

DO

Watch out for local speed limits: each council can set its own.

Make sure you have a full tank before setting out on a drive to the country.

Eat roadkill.

Beware of jam sandwiches in the road – poachers put them out to attract deer in the hope that a driver will knock them over, leaving them some decent roadkill to sell on to the nearest butcher.

DON'T

Throw your rubbish out of the window – I will hunt you down.

Encourage a race with the dogs running out of driveways to chase you.

49

The Only Gay in the Village

Rural Sexuality

'Growing up, I thought I was the only gay in the village.' This is not a line from *Little Britain*'s Daffyd, but a common refrain amongst gay men brought up in the country. Clearly, the Welsh comedy character sounded a chord for many gay people across the land – although it is to be assumed that fewer numbers wear PVC playsuits to the local pub. The traditional image of gays in the country has tended to be either of 'brothers' who run the local village shop, or a rich interior designer/pop star and his boyfriend living in the Big House, tolerated in much the same way as black musicians in the 1930s were tentatively accepted by posh whites: for the entertainment value.

But while the countryside's social fabric may have been slower to catch up with the fast changes emanating from the cities, it is not as far off as is commonly believed. There are pockets of backwardness, of course, but bigotry is as rare in the country as it is in the town.

Statistically, if you are gay you must expect to be in the minority in any village – indeed noticeably so; at least in town there are gay bars where you can enjoy for a few hours the feeling of being in the majority. But that's not to say there aren't any out there. One gay friend of mine told me that as a teenager at school, he was convinced he was alone. But when he moved to London and discovered gay bars, much to his surprise, he bumped into guys he had known when he was growing up. One lesbian couple in Holbeach in Lincolnshire know that they are not the only ones in the village – they have often been told by neighbours about 'ladies like you two' that live down the road, but have found it difficult to find a way to meet them.

The gay men and women I talked to had no stories of violence or aggression against them (although they said they knew of it happening to others), but one said, astutely, 'in the country, they don't say anything, they just blank you'. In an environment where everybody says hello to everybody they pass, whether they know them or not, this in itself can feel pretty isolating.

If you're feeling alone in your gaiety, one solution is to join a sympathetic group, one where you share a sexual preference together with some sort of hobby – for example the Gay Outdoors Club (GOC) or the Gay Caravanning and Camping Club (GCC). Members I spoke to said that the main interest would be the walking or staying in caravans (which, frankly, I find odder than any obscure cult – but there you go, there's something for everyone). But they find relief in being able to be themselves within the group, even if it's just being able to hold hands with their partner when out on a walk.

Moving to a new village, one gay woman wanted to recruit members to the GOC. She tried to put an ad in the local paper but it never made it in – 'they assured me it was just an error and not because the word "gay" was in the copy'. Hmmm. So then she thought she'd put a poster up in the local supermarket. 'I asked the check-out girl if I could put a poster up and she said yes. Then she read it. Twice.' She was unable to look the lesbian in the eye and said the wall was full but she would put it up later (she did). This shyness seems to be the most common reaction that gay men and women are faced with. Many told me of arriving in pubs to be met with a somewhat frosty reaction but later, after a few pints, everyone would get chatting. I have a notion that the shyness is as much about strangers walking into the pub as about them being gay. There is a tiny pub in north rural Yorkshire that is probably still talking about the night 40 gay men and women arrived at once (on a GOC weekend). The regulars turned their backs at first, but by the end of the night, curiosity had got the better of them and everyone was nattering away.

If you are a gay couple moving to a village the advice seems to be to avoid anticipating people's reactions and being on the defensive from the off. They can be sophisticated in the country too. Country people are as likely to find it hard to befriend you if you are just a weekender or don't participate in the village life. Country life does also tend to revolve around family life and the older village inhabitants may not know quite what to say if they can't talk about grandchildren. But if you allow your neighbours to get to know you first, without ever denying who you are, you'll make the friends you want. There is, of course, a smaller pool of people to draw from so you may have to compromise: if the local British Legion invites you to their weekly line-dancing night, you may as well just camp it up and enjoy.

DO

Arrive with an open mind.

Let them get to know the person first – don't be defined by your sexuality.

Join a local group for support when you need it – living in the country can be isolating at times for anyone.

DON'T

Walk about with a red spotted handkerchief in your back left pocket and expect anyone to know what it means.

Invite everyone at the local pub back to yours for pina coladas and a dip in the hot tub – you'll never fit them all in at once.

50

Knowing a Man Who Can

Employing Domestic Staff

Country houses have long been bastions of domestic employment. Before World War II even the middle classes employed several staff: gardener, housekeeper, cook and nanny. The grander houses would also have butlers, ladies' maids, grooms, stable hands, gamekeepers, drivers and footmen – up to 60 fully employed servants would not have been surprising. And all firmly kept below stairs. To a degree, this class/staff ratio still holds, although the middle classes will tend to employ someone who comes in from the village – even if it's just a 'daily'. The upper classes, or the owners of large houses, will most likely have a live-in couple, sharing the jobs between them. The woman will be housekeeper, cook and part-nanny. The man will be gardener, driver, butler and, possibly, gamekeeper.

If you have moved into a grand house the essential thing is to employ locally. Under no circumstances must you move to the country with your favourite Slovakian cleaner. A nanny is perhaps the only employee who can be brought up from town. Secondly, if you find that the previous owners had a cleaner and/or gardener who has worked on the house for many years, you must take them on too – no matter how much they dribble their soup or sit about the place gossiping.

The recent influx of Eastern European workers to Britain has changed the attitude to staff greatly. Once upon a time, even I struggled as to whether I could employ a cleaner for my flat in London, seeing as I was a young, fit girl and read the *Guardian* at least twice a week. (Of course, once the delightful Eva was gainfully employed, for £8 an hour, I quickly settled into the role of Lady of the Manor, or rather, Lady of the Small Flat, leaving bossy notes about cleaning the sink properly and suspecting her of stealing the shampoo.) But lately, as we work longer hours and both parents are often out of the house all day, having 'someone who does' has become increasingly acceptable. With new laws in place regarding minimum wages and holiday entitlements, it is hopefully not too unfair a deal on both sides.

One thing that has changed since ye olden times is the matter of live-in accommodation. Where once a domestic couple would live in a small cottage on the grounds, that is likely to have been rented out to weekending townies for a princely sum. The most likely live-in arrangement for a housekeeper/gardener team will be a studio room above the pig shed.

Individually, in these jobs, they might earn between £25,000 and £30,000 p.a. each. As a couple they are likely to be paid £40,000 in a single pay packet. You might wonder why a husband and wife would squash up together above the swill, earning a modest wage and living largely at the behest of a bossy madam and gruff sir. The answer, according to the employment agencies, is that 'they love the lifestyle. In previous generations they may well have been landowners, or tenants, themselves.' In other words, they still get to live and breathe the country air, work the land, enjoy the comforts of the big house and hold none of the fiscal responsibilities. If everyone gets on well, they are likely to stay in one place for many years, forming a strong bond of loyalty and trust. They are also, however, likely to consider your house and garden as 'theirs'. This can cause problems if, when you buy a house, you take on the previous staff, too. Any plans to change a room's layout or the height of a hedgerow is liable to be fiercely resisted.

If you do employ staff, even part-time, you must register as an employer with your local tax office. If you pay them more than £87 a week, or if they earn more than £87 a week from you and other employers (the onus is on you to find this out) this is essential. There are also various legalities concerning holiday allowance, tax and so on. The real issue with domestic staff is one of gross/net pay. For some reason, with any other job, when told your pay you assume you are being told the gross amount, but domestic staff will assume they are being told the net amount.

It is only fair to be reasonable when it comes to breaks and holiday allowance. In the past staff would be up until the last member or guest of the household had gone to bed, pouring out brandies and standing by the back wall listening to the gossip as small recompense. A grandiose former owner of my grandparents' house in Sussex liked to hold lavish parties. One was themed around a trip on the Titanic, and the gardeners and stable hands were employed to throw buckets of water at the drawing-room windows all night, to give the illusion of being in a storm. I'm not sure he'd get away with it now – at least, not for less than the cost of sending them all on an actual cruise.

Finally, don't expect all your staff to be walking etiquette guides. A daily who comes in to help now and then is liable to pour the white wine into the wrong glass (red wine: large glass; white wine: smaller glass) and stack plates at the table to clear them away. If you mind about this, then you must be clear in advance. Nor do staff tend to wear uniforms any more: Norland nannies, perhaps, but few others. Butlers may wear morning suit trousers but with an ordinary black suit jacket, rather than tails. A housekeeper tends to prefer an attire of jeans and fleece, rather than a starched white apron.

If you are a guest in a house with staff, try not to be awkward about it. Be polite to everybody (there was a horrible snobbery years ago about saying 'thank you' to the butler when he handed you the plate of greens or a Bloody Mary before lunch but I hold no truck with bad manners at *any* time) and don't forget to leave a tip. If you do successfully seduce the maid, however, a tip might be rather an insult.

DO

Clarify whether the pay you are offering is gross or net.

Be reasonable when it comes to breaks and holiday allowance.

Remember your staff at Christmas and make a note of their birthdays.

DON'T

Expect a 'daily' to understand the finer points of service etiquette.

Accuse your staff of stealing the silver unless you are absolutely sure.

51

What to Wear

Getting the Right Kit

What do Kate Moss, Princess Diana and the Duke of Wellington have in common? They have all made the welly a fashion icon in their time. The Duke stepped out in black leather; Princess Diana paved the way for Sloane Rangers in the eighties with their green rubber boots stomping up and down the King's Road; and Mossy grooved at Glastonbury in navy Hunters.

Wellies – or gumboots as the toffs call them – are the first and foremost essential piece of kit for any trip to the country. At almost any time of year, it will be muddy. The rubber wellies we all know and love were first designed and manufactured by the North British Rubber Company in 1955 (now better known as Hunter). First, they invented the shape we know today: moulded around the calf, so the boots don't pull off at the ankle when you get stuck in mud. Second, they made them in green rubber – much more appealing to all the ex-soldiers who'd been wearing black boots during the war. Designed originally for gamekeepers, they were then worn by the estate owners, keen to look like their skilled employees. If you don't want to stick out like a banana in an apple tree, only wear green boots in the country. Red or navy boots are just about acceptable for walks, if worn by incredibly stylish women (e.g. me and my aunt Emma), but black boots are only for mucking out the horses, and anything with rainbow-coloured patterns are best left to a wet day on the high street. Note that La Moss, never known to put a sartorial foot wrong, only ever wears the correctly coloured wellies.

Boots, of course, are only the start of it. Whereas in town anything goes and the more of a rule-breaker you are, the more chic you are, in the country it's all about convention. With Internet shopping, supermarket fashion and endless reams of advice from TV, newspapers and magazines on what to wear, even those in the country are catching up with their urbanite cousins. But few would break the rules completely; they prefer merely to tweak them.

So what are the rules? First off, clothes must look as if they have been chosen for practicality rather than style. A skirt may have a pattern or flourish on it, but will also be warm. A jacket could have a stylish cut but will be waterproof. It's recently become a lot easier to combine your fashion nous with worsted since the advent of the Really Wild Clothing Company and Eric Clapton took over Cordings. Plus, of course, everyone from Vivienne Westwood to George at Asda has done a little fashioning in tweed. Even the Game Fair, a large county fair where rural folk get together to meet and buy their farm and field sport equipment, has started to plan catwalk shows – something no one would have predicted from the days when moth-eaten cashmere jumpers and grandpa's flat cap were the only *de rigueur* items in the country.

Avoid wearing black in the country. It is just about acceptable in the evenings, but only for a formal supper or dinner and dance. Perhaps the yokels can never quite shake off their instinct for camouflage but the only colours worn are brown, green, muddy yellows, pale golds, bronzes, cream, dusty pinks and maybe a dash of red. There is also an instinct to resist looking as if any real effort has been made. A beautiful dress will be covered up with a long cardigan, or a fitted suit will be accessorised with badly scuffed shoes. No man's clothes should ever look crisp and clean: if you must buy a new walking jacket, drag it in some mud and leave it outside for a night in the rain before wearing it. Holes in socks (if not in jumpers), elbow patches and a slight smell of mothballs are all acceptable accessories.

In the morning, for breakfast, always come down fully dressed but not yet with the costume flourishes that you are saving for lunch (i.e. no jewellery or plus twos). Be ready to swap shoes for boots and don waxed coats, long scarves and caps for a mid-morning walk. Lunch means a quick wash and brush-up (of yourself not the dogs), and I would wear something warm – most dining-rooms in the country are freezing. Generally one wears the same thing all day and night and preferably three days in a row but in the smarter houses you need to change for dinner (see chapter 54).

194

Even then, of course, it's not that simple. A fashion writer for the *Mail on Sunday* got it right when she quoted a 'fabulously astute country bystander' who told her it's not Barbour but Schoffel, not Hunter but Le Chameau and not wet Labrador but lurcher or border terrier. Bang on. And you can identify me as a TIC (townie in the country) in seconds because I can be seen wearing red Hunter boots to my local village every Saturday morning. My boyfriend (for whom a roll in the hay is something pleasant and for me brings on an allergy attack) wears walking shoes everywhere unless extremely muddy. Even then, his only gumboots are black and cost £7.99 from the local garage. While I am sitting in a Wiltshire kitchen as I write this, dressed in a long brown corduroy skirt, he is quite happily sitting on the sofa in black jeans. If you're from the country you do what the hell you like: townies have to try a bit harder. And in trying harder we look all wrong. Some games in life simply can't be won.

DO

Wear any colour that makes you think of autumn.

Wear your riding kit to a nightclub in town.

Wear wellies to the village shop if you want to look like a townie.

Leave your new clobber out in the elements for a night or two.

DON'T

Fight the temptation to wear the same clothes several days running and belt your trousers up with string.

52

Adult Entertainment

Dinner Party Games

Go for supper at a friend's house in Birmingham, Edinburgh or Nottingham and the evening is likely to be rounded off by a glass of brandy, perhaps a cigar if the hosts are really pushing the boat out, and maybe a small tiff with your spouse before shuffling into a taxi home. In the country it's a different matter altogether – for a start, you are most likely there for the whole night until the morning. In other words, you will be effectively trapped into doing what the hosts want to do. And if you're staying with someone exceptionally vibrant and sociable, (a.k.a. irritating), like me, you'll hear these terrifying words after port and coffee: 'Now, let the games begin!'

As with most activities in the country, games are a mere ruse for flirtation. 'Sardines' is the best for this – one person runs off to hide and everyone else has to find them. When you find them, you hide with them, squashing up nose to nose (like sardines in a tin – geddit?) and the loser is the last one to discover the dark corner. As a small child I found this game quite alarming – not least because if I was third to find the hiding place, the two grown-ups already there would not be best pleased to have a nine-year-old girl disturb their frolics.

There's really only one rule when it comes to games in a country house – you absolutely, completely and utterly have to join in. Paradoxically, you mustn't really mind about winning or losing, without being totally apathetic either way. Highly competitive types who elbow everyone else out of the way or get red-faced when telling team mates what to do just look ridiculous. Similarly, the one who has no spirit of competition at all and never minds if they are out of the game immediately is equally tiresome. The only way through it is to drink – a lot – and get louder and more amusing (if only to yourself) until the hosts bore of their gaming guests and send everyone off to bed.

If as a townie you get caught in this maelstrom, the most effective way to blend in and gain some (Brownie) points, is to have a game or two of your own up your sleeve. At the very least you should know how to play them, as by the time 14 bottles of wine have been drunk no one will be capable of pointing you in the right direction for the loo, let alone explain the rules of a game.

THE GAME

The classic country game is called simply 'The Game', although many mistakenly call it charades. Those of you who were members of The Lionel Blair Fan Club will remember his consummate skill in television's *Give Us A Clue*, which followed the same rules as The Game.

Divide everyone up into two teams and put them in separate rooms. Each team then comes up with a number of titles of books, films, plays, songs and musicals, and writes them on scraps of paper, which are then put into a hat. The hats are swapped between the teams. Once you are all back in the same room and have stopped squabbling over the comfiest armchair, one member of a team pulls a title out and must then act it out, in silence and without props, to his team who try to guess what he's doing. The winning team is the one that guesses the most titles correctly.

There are some basic mimes: First you must indicate whether the title is a book (motion palms out, like a book opening), film (mime an old-fashioned cine camera), play (mime stage curtains) or song (jazz hands).

Next show how many words the title contains by holding up the appropriate number of fingers.

To show which word you are acting out, hold up your first, second or fourth finger, etc.

Then mime whatever is necessary to get your team to work out what the title is. If you want to mime a word that *sounds* like the one in the title, grab your earlobe between finger and thumb and wriggle your earlobe. Or you can break a word up into syllables (show the number of syllables of the words by placing the same number of fingers on your upper arm). Holding out your thumb and forefinger as a small box indicates connecting words (in, to, of, at, and) and the shape of a 'T' with your fingers means the word 'the'. To show your team mates that they have guessed a word correctly, put one finger on your nose and point another finger at them.

Much hilarity ensues.

IN THE MANNER OF THE WORD

This is the good one to have up your sleeve as not everyone knows it but it is always a big hit. One person is sent out of the room and everyone else must settle on an adverb: e.g. 'boringly', 'slowly', 'romantically, 'over-enthusiastically' and so on. The person comes back in the room and picks someone out to do a task – say, making coffee, painting a picture or combing their hair – 'in the manner of the word'. So they must proceed to paint a picture over-enthusiastically, or whatever. Inevitably there is a temptation to start making up adverbs that hint at an in-joke ('Georgina-ishly', 'frumpishly') and it's all terribly funny. Especially when drunk.

DO

Join in at full throttle.

Keep topping up everyone's drinks.

Tell the object of your affections where you'll be hiding so they can find you first.

DON'T

Care terribly about winning but do mind a bit about losing.

Tell the children to go to bed when the games begin.

Lock yourself in the loo for the duration of the escapades.

53

Playing Lord of the Manor

How to be the Perfect Host

OK, so you've bought the country pile, you've planted the roses round the door, admired the view of leaping lambs in the field opposite and written 'peace and quiet' in your diary for every day until 2033. But there's a problem. All those pesky townies you mortgaged yourself to the hilt to escape will be on the telephone angling for an invitation.

Having friends to stay in the country is not the same as a quick supper in your flat, ten minutes away from a Tube stop. First off, give them clear directions down the winding lanes to your abode – country people usually give instructions that don't include any road names (there aren't any), just landmarks, which can't be seen at night in the driving rain. Nearly everyone gets lost or trains are delayed, so cook stew not soufflé for the Friday night in case you have to drive halfway back to the city to fetch them. Saturdays in the country are all about long walks, or going to the local point-to-point. Stock the house with plenty of spare wellies (the green kind) as someone's girlfriend is bound to arrive in her Jimmy Choo ballet pumps. Wellies tend to go walkies, so put your name in them (or the house name, if you're very grand) and count them before people leave on Sunday. Also make it clear that your guests must remove their boots by the back door after the walk. Pick a walk: choosing preferably one with a pub *en route*. But make sure it's one where the locals won't be irritated by a pack of loud townies chasing local ale with tequila.

Saturday night suppers in the country are traditionally dinner party affairs, with townie friends and country neighbours thrown in together. Country people seem to talk of little else besides the sex lives of their dog, sheep or neighbours and relish the townie stories of rumpus in nightclubs. Encourage your urban friends to talk about their latest escapades at London's Boujis or Twisted Elegance in Manchester.

Sundays are for hangovers, newspapers, brunch and a late Sunday roast. If the papers aren't delivered (and they rarely are out in the sticks) then you'll have to drive to the village to get them: buy two sets to save any scrabbling over the colour supplements. Present them all with a vat of Bloody Mary. Then save yourself some hassle and take everyone back to the local pub for a late lunch. The perfect guest leaves just after teatime. If anyone threatens to overstay their welcome all you have to do is tell them the manure is being delivered soon and they'd better get their car out of the driveway.

DO

Give your guests clear directions.

Have a plan for the weekend – walk, games, orgy, whatever.

Remember to get two sets of newspapers for Sunday brunch.

Give your guests VERY clear instructions if you have a burglar alarm.

DON'T

Hesitate to encourage a row between townie and country friends – it's always fun to watch fireworks.

54

Bread and Butter

How to be the Perfect Guest

Rich people all over the world know there's only one accessory that truly glorifies their sky-high credit limits: a whacking great pile in the country. Which can be good news for the rest of us minions – we might get invited to stay for the weekend.

Not everyone in the countryside is posh but big house owners like to show off their lord of the manor status by imposing old-fashioned rules on their guests. Follow my advice and you can spend the rest of your Sundays pampered in style by a roaring log fire, with a Labrador at your feet.

First of all, turn up when you say you will – preferably about 8 p.m. on a Friday night. Stumbling drunkenly off the last train to Malmesbury won't bode well for the rest of your stay. Be sure, too, to check the pronunciation of the station you are alighting at (how is anyone to know that Ingatestone is 'Insnesher'?).

To be on the safe side, pack something smart for Saturday night, plus comfy trousers and cardigans in varying shades of green and brown (take absolutely nothing in black if you are staying with toffs). Do pack carefully if you're staying somewhere frightfully grand – they might have a butler unpack your case for you. And be careful what you leave out on the bed or on the nightstand – hostesses tend to take guests on tours of the house and your condom packets will be fuel for gossip. One good tip: pack an extra jumper to wear at night as country house bedrooms are invariably freezing. My uncle once had to put on his bed every single thing that wasn't actually nailed to the floor, including all the bath towels and a large Persian rug. I also like to take a slab of chocolate rather than raid the kitchen when I get hungry – in huge houses with too many guests and too small portions of supper, one almost always does. As a general rule, all guests should stay out of the kitchen – all hostesses hate anyone to see the mess and chaos that prevails behind the scenes.

Arrive with a decent present for your host: a potted plant or a sumptuous box of chocolates. Avoid hand-tied bouquets, no matter how pretty. No hostess wants to be struggling with scissors and cellophane when she's trying to show everyone to their rooms. If you leave it to the last minute and the shops are shut, it's better to take nothing at all and send something later. On no account turn up with a soggy bunch of carnations from the petrol station. Toffs tend not to like presents at all, and will almost never take them to friends' houses, but they should accept well chosen alcohol or delectable food with good grace.

As a guest, the key thing to remember at all times

is that you have surrendered all rights to do things the way you want to from the moment you cross the threshold. As a human being you have fewer rights than you would retain as a guest in the dingiest hotel, where at least the payment of a bill entitles you to make some demands. As your host's guest, you eat when everyone else eats, drink only when they drink and join in enthusiastically with all planned activities. Perhaps, given the choice, you would rather eat your ear-wax than talk to the local vicar before lunch. No one cares.

Saturday morning should be reasonably relaxed. If it is a large party, say a shooting weekend, breakfast will be held in the dining-room. Whether you are in a grand house or tiny cottage, help yourself to whatever the host has put out. This might be cereal or the full monty, slowly congealing in silver platters kept barely warm by a burning tea light beneath. Get down early, I say. Never wear your dressing-gown outside your bedroom, no matter how silky or smart. Keep it casual: a heavily made-up face can put the other guests off their eggs.

After breakfast is a good time to get yourself out from under your hostess's feet and you can have a quick walk (you can always offer to take the dogs out) or read the papers. A stay in the country can feel like just one long chain of food-related events – I once put on a stone staying with my grandparents for a week – so you may as well get some movement in where you can. Soon it will be lunch and not long after that, tea with hot buttered toast and maybe some fruitcake. A quick bath to follow, perhaps, and everyone is ready for supper.

A little aside – if your hosts are proper nobs, their rules are slightly different. I mention them here because while there are a diminishing number of very posh people who insist on Edwardian manners, those that do are fairly fierce about it. I will lay their rules down here – and then you can choose to ignore them.

Saturday night is party night. The toffs (or show-offs) will insist on black tie – at the very least, they will change for dinner. There may be several courses – just follow the old rule of using the cutlery from the outside in. Just one caveat at the posh pads: only use your fork for pudding. One woman I know can eat custard with just a fork. There will be a different wine for each course, which you are not obliged to finish or even drink. Just don't refuse it – few things are more annoying to a nob than someone refusing alcohol. Talk to the person on your left for the starter, and to the right for the main (or follow the direction of your host). Pudding comes before cheese, and finally out comes the port.

Port is the moment that divides the Old Posh from the New Posh. There are a few households left where the women will leave the supper table to have coffee in the drawing-room, while the men drink the port. You can call this sexist if you like, but actually your host is likely to be secretly thrilled at the row if you insist on making a scene about it. If you stay – man or woman – the port passes to the left, even if the only person taking a refill is sitting on your right.

Just one last point about the nobs: don't put on a

posh accent. They'll see straight through it and it will only delight a snob and infuriate a liberal. Got all that? Now ignore it.

Once you've tottered up to bed replete with your repast there's just the little matter of the small room. Bathroom etiquette is a peculiarity of country houses as few of them have locks – the general thinking is that there are enough to go round to have one assigned per bedroom, but this isn't always the case. If the water isn't running, sing to yourself to keep intruders at bay. Be careful not to use all the hot water as even the grandest houses have a limited supply, and if your partner gets in before you, you're going to have to bathe in lukewarm grey water: it's still better than cold clean water.

Most houses in the country cannot function without domestic staff – either several servants or a 'daily' who 'does', coming in to change the bedsheets and peel the potatoes. Even if you don't see any staff, you need to leave a tip in your bedroom at the end of the weekend – about a fiver per person per night is right. Even if no one was employed, the hostess will be pleased that you thought the weekend was run with the sort of efficiency that only a Jeeves could muster. And after all, the cost of the tip is still cheaper than the best deal at Travelodge and you will probably drink a lot more Château Lafite. Remember to write a charming thank you letter the second you get home (e-mail or, horror, text messaging, simply will not do). This is known as a 'bread-and-butter' letter – presumably because, as the guest, you're the one who is jammy.

DO

Turn up when you say you will.

Pack something warm to wear at night.

Stay out of the kitchen at all times.

DON'T

Refuse invitations to go for a walk/join in a game/watch a film.

Tear articles and less still, whole pages, out of the newspapers.

Put on a fake posh accent.

55

Contagious Concerns

Countryside Scares

Even in times of beautiful sunshine, there will always be townies resistant to the idea of going to the countryside and if they read the papers, I can't really blame them. Foot-and-mouth disease (FMD), bird flu and blue-tongue disease have been making recent appearances, and the memory of mad cow disease is not yet dim. Coupled with the increasing risk of flooding (less global warming; more bad planning and drainage), a mini-break in Afghanistan probably holds more appeal. But don't be put off: now, more than ever, it is crucial that the countryside remains open and townies continue to enjoy the golden fields that lie beyond.

To be clear, it is perfectly safe to go to the countryside. FMD does not affect humans – the last person to be infected was in 1966. In fact, in most other countries around the world, cattle are riddled with FMD; it is highly likely that you have had hundreds of burgers, steaks and sausages, which have been injected with the FMD vaccine. But because the EU enjoys FMD-free status, there is a somewhat hysterical response to the disease in this country. Infected cattle may even recover, and it could be argued that slaughter of the diseased animals is needless, except that not to kill them would mean it spreads and all British cattle would be banned from export to anywhere within the EU, meaning the loss of millions of pounds to already struggling farmers.

Farmers are unsentimental about their animals – you won't find sheep curled up on the armchair, or cows decorated with pink ribbons – but they care deeply for them, taking pride in their health and strength. One farmer I know in Hampshire, just a few miles south of a briefly excluded zone in Surrey during a recent scare, has a 'closed herd', which he has nurtured for nearly 40 years. They are pure breeds, producing the finest milk, and should he have to slaughter them, his entire life's work would go up in flames.

After the burning pyres of 2001, villagers rallied round and created farmers' markets (see chapter 2), as a way of helping farmers sell produce and restore bonds with their customers. So keep going to your local market and buying local produce – all the food is perfectly safe to eat and it's vital that we do not lose the trust that has been so carefully and successfully built up over the last few years.

Just for quick reference: bird flu does of course hold a danger for humans once caught, but while the threat has been hanging about for some time in Britain, it has failed to materialise on the scale promised by the tabloids. You can be sure that no one wants it to disappear more than the farmers do and every precaution will be taken by them to ensure this. Blue-tongue disease is not especially attractive (ever eaten a biro?) but nor is it radically dangerous. The resultant malaises (reproductive problems, congenital defects, ulcers, etc.) are highly disputed by scientists, and only occur after persistent infection. In any case, a hard frost can kill off the carriers (which are mere gnats, blown over from Europe).

The floods are not good – they may get worse. I don't mean to be trite, but I would suggest you buy a house on a hill. (OK, I do mean to be a bit trite, but unless the planners and insurance people sort it out, there's not a lot you can do.)

In writing this book, I exhort you to go to the countryside, and I hope when you get there you see what I mean by the beauty and the peace of the land. Without the countryside working, nothing works. Support your countrymen: go for a roll in the hay.

DO

Keep supporting your farmers – go to your local farmers' market.

Take any precautions you are asked to (sterilising boots, avoiding exclusion zones).

DON'T

Go to the butchers wearing your grandfather's World War II gas mask.

Feed blue biros to the cows to create a false alarm, no matter how hilarious.

Stop going to the countryside.

Directory

(Useful websites and telephone numbers.
See: www.mudandthecity.com for links.)

SPRING

Riding

British Horse Society: www.bhs.org.uk
An equestrian charity, with masses of leaflets available on care for your horse, *Highway Code*, etc. Also a nationwide list of approved livery stables.

Pony Club: www.pcuk.org

Farmers' Markets

Find certified farmers' markets around the country: www.farmersmarkets.net

Antiques

For a comprehensive listing of all antique fairs month-by-month around the country: www.antiquecollectors guide.co.uk

Hotspots:

Honiton, Devon – around 30 antique shops in the town: www.honitonantiques.co.uk

Tetbury, Gloucestershire: www.tetbury.org

Tetsworth, Oxfordshire – The Swan is a marketplace and restaurant, which holds 40 rooms of fine antiques: www.theswan.co.uk

Long Melford, Suffolk – *Lovejoy* was filmed here and there are streets of antique shops, plus lots of other independent boutiques: www.longmelford.co.uk

Stately Homes

The National Trust: www.nationaltrust.org.uk For everything on the National Trust – houses, gardens, events.

To recreate the look of a stately home in your own two-bed flat, buy original materials from: www.countryhouseantiquetextiles.co.uk

Badminton

Badminton Horse Trials: 0870 2423436; www.badminton-horse.co.uk

Other premier equestrian events:

Burghley Horse Trials: www.burghley-horse.co.uk

Blenheim International Horse Trials: www.blenheim-horse.co.uk

Royal Windsor Horse Show: www.royal-windsor-horse-show.co.uk

Hen and Stag Weekends

To rent a house:
Rural Retreats: 01386 701177; www.ruralretreats.co.uk
The Big House Company: 01823 662673; www.thebig
houseco.com
Call of the Wild: 01639 700388; www.callofthe
wild.co.uk
Organises full-on activity-packed weekends in Wales,
but you stay in B&Bs, rather than your own rented
cottage.

SUMMER

Car Boot Sales

For regular listings of car boot sales, register for 12
months for a small fee at: www.carbootcalendar.com

Camping

Find your site:
www.happycampers.co.uk
www.caravancampingsites.co.uk
www.ukcampsite.co.uk
www.campinguk.com

Kit:
www.armytents.co.uk
www.tents-direct.co.uk
www.millets.co.uk

Fishing

For a National Rod Licence: www.environment-agency. gov.uk/subjects/fish

Fishing gear:
Real Tree: www.realtree.com
Get kitted out in this US hunting brand; usually pretty trendy with young fishermen.
Farlows: www.farlows.co.uk
Find the traditional country sportswear at Farlows, Pall Mall, London W1.

Check for fishing on canals through local tourist offices.

Ascot

For more information and tickets, go to: www.ascot.co.uk

Croquet

Croquet sets from www.croquetonline.co.uk (Jaques is the original and best maker of the game).

Official rules from the Croquet Association: www. croquet.org.uk

Fêtes

Check local tourist offices for notices of village fêtes.

Recommended:
Shellingford Fête, Shellingford Community Hall, Oxfordshire: www.fernham.info/events.html
St Martin's Green Fête, Knebworth: www.knebworth.org

Snitterfield Village Fête, Warwickshire: www.snitterfield.com

Heydour Parish Midsummer Fête, Heydour Parish Millennium Green, Aisby, Lincolnshire: www.grantham-online.co.uk

Wicken Fête and Dog Show, Wicken, Cambridgeshire: www.wicken-village.org.uk

Radley Village Fête & Flower Show, Radley, Oxfordshire: www.radleyvillage.org.uk

Polo

Veuve Clicquot Gold Cup Final, Cowdray Park, Sussex: www.cowdraypolo.co.uk

Cartier International Polo, Guards Polo Club, Windsor: www.guardspoloclub.com

For rules and regulations, see Hurlingham Polo Association: www.hpa-polo.co.uk

Vineyards

Ridgeview Estate, Sussex: www.ridgeview.co.uk
Breaky Bottom, Sussex: www.breaky-bottom.co.uk
Wyken Vineyard, Suffolk: www.wyken-vineyards.co.uk
Stanlake Park Wine Estate, Berkshire: www.stanlakepark.com

Cowes Week

For all you need to know: www.skandiacowesweek.co.uk

Reports on: www.yachtingworld.com

Listen to the racing commentary and interviews on Cowes Radio: 87.7FM

Getting there – at Southampton, take the fast Red Jet catamaran to Cowes. See www.redfunnel.co.uk

Country Rocks

Countryside Rocks: www.countryside-alliance.org

Various stately homes (Petworth House in Sussex or Blickling Hall in Norfolk, for example) host rock concerts during the summer. See: www.nationaltrust.org.uk

West Wycombe Music Festival, Bucks: www.classic fantastic.co.uk

Picnic Concerts as arranged by English Heritage. Venues are: Audley End House, Essex; Marble Hill, Twickenham; and Battle Abbey, Sussex: www.picnicconcerts.com

Buy a shooting stick so you can take a pew wherever you are: www.sticks-etc.co.uk

Literary Festivals

Aldeburgh Literary Festival, Suffolk: 01728 452389; www.aldeburghbookshop.co.uk
Bath Literature Festival: www.bathlitfest.org.uk
Sunday Times Oxford Literary Festival: www.sunday times-oxfordliteraryfestival.co.uk
Hay Festival, Wales: www.hayfestival.com

Surfing, Windsurfing and Sailing

Datchet Watersports, just outside Windsor: 01753 683990; www.datchetwsports.force9.co.uk
Sailing and windsurfing courses available.

Bray Lake, Windsor: www.braylake.com
For windsurfing and sailing.

Newquay, Cornwall. All the info you need on finding hotels, surf-cam, tide times, etc. www.surfnewquay.co.uk

West Wittering, Chichester: www.westwitteringbeach.co.uk

Learn the lingo: www.surfing-waves.com/surf_talk.htm

Golf

Best golf clubs with relaxing clubhouses:
Goodwood, Chichester, West Sussex: 01243 755144; www.goodwood.co.uk/golf
Stoke Park Club, Stoke Poges, Bucks: 01753 71717; www.stokeparkclub.com/golf
The Grove, Chandler's Cross, Hertfordshire: 01923 294266; www.thegrove.co.uk

Garden Operas

Grange Park Opera, near Winchester, Hampshire: 01962 868888; www.grangeparkopera.com
Glyndebourne Festival Opera, near Lewes, East Sussex: 01273 813813; www.glyndebourne.com
Garsington Opera, near Oxford: 01865 361636

Opera at llford, near Bath, Somerset: 01225 868124
Longborough Festival Opera, near Moreton-in-Marsh,
Gloucestershire: 01451 830292
Hever Castle, Edenbridge, Kent: 01732 866114;
www.heverlakeside.co.uk

Look out for dates by The Garden Opera Company:
www.gardenopera.co.uk

Coastal Gourmet

East Beach Cafe, Littlehampton, Sussex: www.eastbeach
cafe.co.uk
The Shed, Porthgain, Wales: 01348 831518; www.
theshedporthgain.co.uk
Hive Beach Cafe, Burton Bradstock, Dorset: 01308
897070; www.hivebeachcafe.co.uk
The Victoria, Park Road, Holkham, Norfolk: 01328
713230; www.holkham.co.uk
Whitstable Oyster Fishery Company, Whitstable, Kent:
01227 276856; www.oysterfishery.co.uk
Rick Stein's Seafood Restaurant, Riverside, Padstow,
Cornwall: 01841 53Z700; www.rickstein.com

AUTUMN

Walking

Ramblers Association: www.ramblers.org.uk
For right of way maps and good routes.

For a fee, download step-by-step guides to 3,500 walks
around Britain: www.walkingworld.com

DIRECTORY

Heritage Open Days

www.heritageopendays.org

Clay Shoots

Royal Berkshire Shooting School: 01491 672900;
www.rbss.co.uk
Lessons from £55; one-on-one £79. Cartridges and
clays paid for separately.

Purdeys (the traditional outfitters): www.purdey.com
Get all your kit here first.

Country Club UK: www.countryclubuk.com/gunroom
For general info on shooting schools in the UK and
hotels to stay at with shooting.

Mushrooming

(Be extra careful if you go shrooming.)

Good woods for fungi forays:
New Forest, Hampshire (www.forestry.gov.uk)
Rendlesham Forest, Suffolk
Alice Holt Woodland Park, Surrey
Hamsterley Forest, Durham

Fruit Picking

Find a pick-your-own farm: www.pick-your-own.org.uk

Apple Day is held in October. See: www.common
ground.org.uk for details of national events.

Advice on collection, germination and nurturing seeds, from: www.treecouncil.org.uk

Deer Rutting

Where to see the rutting:
Many National Trust parks, including Attingham, near Shrewsbury; Belton, near Grantham, Lincolnshire; Charlecote; near Warwick; Dinefwr in Carmarthenshire; and Lyme, (near Stockport, Cheshire.

See: www.nationaltrust.org.uk

Perfect Pubs

Alastair Sawday guide books are recommended: www.sawdays.co.uk

Halloween

Various stately homes stage Halloween events. Check out: Blenheim Palace, Oxford: 08700 602080; www.blenheimpalace.com
Somerleyton Hall, Suffolk: 01502 730224; www.somerleyton.co.uk
Traquair House, Peebleshire: 01896 830323; www.traquair.co.uk
Kentwell Hall, Suffolk: 01787 310207; www.kentwell.co.uk
Escot Park, Devon: 07814 036634; www.escot-devon.co.uk

Check various National Trust houses: www.national
trust.org.uk

Bonfire Night

Find a procession through the local tourist office websites

Recommended:
Torchlit procession in Battle, Sussex: www.battle
bonfire.co.uk
Several different processions begin in Lewes, East Sussex:
www.lewesbonfirecouncil.org.uk
Ottery St Mary tar barrels: www.tarbarrels.co.uk

WINTER

Jumps Season

Ascot Racecourse, Ascot, Berkshire: 08707 227227;
www.ascot.co.uk

Kempton Park, Sunbury-on-Thames, Middlesex: 01932
78229292; www.kempton.co.uk
Holds the King George VI Chase on Boxing Day.

Sandown Park, Esher, Surrey: 01372 464348; www.
sandown.co.uk
The William Hill-Tingle Creek chase jumps are the
hot ticket.

Cheltenham Racecourse, Cheltenham, Gloucestershire:
1242 513014; www.cheltenham.co.uk
The Festival (mid-March) is the equivalent of the

Olympics for jumps. There are four days and they have begun to hold a Ladies' Day, so dust off the hats.

For full details on all fixtures, see: www.britishhorse racing.com

Hunting

To find your local meet: www.mfha.org.uk

Point-to-Points

For details and fixture dates, see: www.pointopoint.co.uk

Talking Point: 09068 446061. The sport's contact number for going, time of meeting and doubtful weather.

Winter Beaches

Whitstable, Kent
Famous for its oysters and Tracey Emin's beach hut. Eat at The Whitstable Oyster Fishery Restaurant – booking in advance strongly recommended: 01227 276856; www.oysterfishery.co.uk
The Hotel Continental has eight specially converted beach huts on the beach that you can stay in: 01227 280280; www.hotelcontinental.co.uk

The Isle of Purbeck, Dorset
This beautiful stretch of Jurassic coast is the only World Heritage Site in the UK. Take the Swanage steam train from Corfe Castle to get there: www.swanagerailway.co.uk

Pleasure piers
If you get your fun from pleasure piers, there are 55 around the country. See: www.piers.co.uk

For traditional seaside nostalgia, see: www.seasidehistory. co.uk

Christmas Fairs

Tatton Park, Knutsford, Cheshire: 01625 534400; www.tattonpark.org.uk

Bath Christmas Market: 01225 396417
Wooden chalets showcase Bath's independent retailers, with hand-made crafts, decorations and toys.

Langport Christmas Market, Somerset: 01458 253527
Stalls with presents, mulled wine and mince pies.

Arty Weekends

Shakespeare's houses (the cottage he grew up in, his wife Anne Hathaway's cottage and others): 01789 201806/836; www.shakespeare.org.uk

The Bronte Birthplace, Thornton, Yorkshire: 01274 830849; www.brontebirthplace.org.uk This is where the three sisters, Charlotte, Emily and Anne, lived with their parents as small girls, from 1815 until 1820. Restored to the Regency period by its current owners, visiting is by arrangement only.

Bronte Parsonage Museum, Haworth, West Yorkshire: 01535 642323; www.bronte.org.uk

This is where the famous books were written and *Jane Eyre* was first imagined by Charlotte.
Bridge Cottage, Flatford, East Bergholt, Suffolk: 01206 298260; www.nationaltrust.org.uk
Houses a permanent collection of Constable sketches and an exhibition on the artist.

The World of Beatrix Potter, Bowness-on-Windermere, Cumbria: www.hop-skip-jump.com
A dedicated centre to the creatures of Peter Rabbit and co. Or you can walk around the shores of Lake Windermere, through wooded fells and the villages of Sawrey and Hawkshead, all of which inspired Miss Potter.

Fowey Hall Hotel, Fowey, Cornwall: 01726 833866; www.foweyhallhotel.co.uk
The *Wind in the Willows* author Kenneth Grahame was inspired by holidays spent at Fowey, Cornwall. The Fowey Hall Hotel claims to be the original 'Toad Hall' and the Wild Wood is close by, known in real life as Ethy Woods, on the banks of the River Fowey, which the hotel overlooks.

Snowdrops

Anglesey Abbey, Lode, Cambridge, Cambridgeshire: 01223 811200.
More than 100 varieties on show in this 100-acre garden.

Belton House, Grantham, Lincolnshire: 01476 566116.

Snowdrop displays in the grounds of a seventeenth-century country house.

Kingston Lacy, Wimborne Minster, Dorset: 01202 883402.

Colesbourne Park, halfway between Cirencester and Cheltenham: 01242 870264.

For more details on these and lots of other snowdrop displays as well as guided snowdrop walks, see: www.nationaltrust.org.uk

Scottish Snowdrop Festival: white.visitscotland.com/snowdrops

Buy bulbs from:
The Snowdrop Company: 01993 842177.
Avon Bulbs: 01460 242177; www.avonbulbs.co.uk

Pancake Day

Check tourist offices for local events.

Norwich Cathedral Pancake Race is a race between the choir boys. 'Flailing flurries of fabric' guaranteed: 01603 213300; www.cathedral.org.uk

PERENNIALS

Buying a Cottage

Search for properties on: www.countrylife.co.uk; www.savills.co.uk; www.knightfrank.co.uk; www.struttand parker.com; www.carterjonas.co.uk

Dogs

The countryside code on controlling your dog: www.codcefngwlad.org.uk/dog.htm

Since 2004, new laws have marked 'access land' on open countryside, moors, heath and down. Dog owners may walk with their dogs off the lead except between March 1 and July 31. See: www.countrysideaccess.gov.uk for maps.

How much is that doggie in the window?:
Greyhound and Lurcher Rescue: www.greyhound andlurcherrescue.co.uk
Dog rescue, with pages for breed contacts: www.dogpages.org.uk
Dogs Trust: www.dogstrust.org.uk

To find a hotel that welcomes dogs: www.dogstrust.org.uk/information/dogfriendlyvenues

Dating

The County Register Ltd: 020 8994 8222; www.the countyregister.com

Just Woodland Friends: (also Autumn Friends): 0845 370 8180; www.justwoodlandfriends.com
Walking and friendship for 40s-70.

Horse & Country Singles: www.horseandcountrysingles. com

The Country Bureau: 01452 614858; www.thecountry bureau.com

Muddy Matches: www.muddymatches.co.uk

Countryside Love: www.countryside-love.co.uk

Partners4farmers: www.partners4farmers.com

Love Horse: www.lovehorse.co.uk

Keeping Chickens

Eglu Hen Parties: www.omlet.com
Buy a hen coop, and you can sign up for a short course on how to rear chickens.

Gay in the Village

Gay Caravan & Camping Club: www.gaycaravanclub. com

To find a walking club near you: Gay Outdoors Club: www.goc.org.uk

Country-wide events: www.outeverywhere.com

Find gay people in your area: www.gaydar.com

Staff

See the classified section of *Country Life* for domestic staff agencies.

What to Wear

The original green rubber welly: www.hunterboots.com

Le Chameau boots are leather lined and very smart: www.lechameau.com

Perfect Host

Pretend to be lord or lady of the manor; Cottages/mansions to rent for the weekend or longer:
www.thewowhousecompany.com
www.blandings.co.uk
www.uniquehomestays.com/whatisuhs.asp

Calendar

SPRING

March

1   Brown trout season opens
14 Coarse fishing season closes
    Cheltenham National Hunt Festival
    Flat Racing season opens

April

East Anglian Game and Country Fair
Grand National Steeplechase, Aintree
Craven Meeting, Newmarket, Suffolk
Spring Meeting, Newbury, Berkshire
Whitbread Gold Cup, Sandown Park Racecourse,
Esher, Surrey
Harrogate Spring Flower Show, Harrogate, Yorkshire
Royal Shakespeare Company Theatre season opens,
Stratford-on-Avon, Gloucestershire

May

Badminton Horse Trials
Royal Windsor Horse Show
Chatsworth Horse Trials
Balmoral Show
Devon County Show
Glyndebourne Festival opens
Highclere Country Fair
Royal Bath and West Show
Polo season starts
The Guineas Meeting, Newmarket, Suffolk
Chester Races, The Roodee, Chester, Cheshire
Newbury International Spring Meeting
Marlborough Cup Race
The Guardian Hay Festival
Bath International Music Festival

SUMMER

June

16 Coarse fishing season opens
Ascot
East of England County Show
Sussex Game Fair
Royal Highland Show
Royal Norfolk Show
Aldeburgh Festival of Music and the Arts
Royal Cornwall Show
Goodwood Festival of Speed

Ludlow Festival

July

Garsington Manor Opera
Henley Royal Regatta
Royal Show, Stoneleigh Park, Warwickshire
Game Conservancy Scottish Fair
Great Yorkshire Show
Kent County Show
World Snail Racing Championships, Norfolk
Veuve Clicquot Gold Cup Final
Royal Welsh Show
CLA Game Fair
Cartier International Polo Tournament
Grange Park Opera Festival
Cheltenham International Festival of Music
Royal Welsh Show
Peterborough Hound Show
Glorious Goodwood

August

12   Grouse season begins (The Glorious Twelfth)
Taunton Flower Show
Festival of British Eventing, Gatcombe
Cowes Week
British Birdwatching Fair
York Races
Cowal Highland Gathering
Chatsworth Country Fair
World Bog Snorkelling, Wales

AUTUMN

September

1   Partridge season begins
    Burghley Horse Trials
    Braemar Royal Highland Gathering
    Blenheim Horse Trials
    Royal Berkshire Show
    Windsor Horse Driving Trials
    National Trust Autumn Plant Sale

October

1   Pheasant shooting season begins
31 Salmon fishing season ends
31 Brown trout season ends
31 Halloween
    National Ploughing Championships
    National Apple Day
    Deer rutting begins
    Horse of the Year Show
    Cheltenham Festival of Literature

November

1   Hunting and Point to Point season opens
5   Guy Fawkes Day
    Paddy Power Gold Cup, Cheltenham – traditionally opens the jumps season

WINTER

December

10 Grouse season ends
25 Christmas Day
26 Boxing Day Meeting – King George VI chase at Kempton Park Racecourse
26 Boxing Day meets – local hunts nationwide

January

15 Salmon fishing season begins (depending on the river)
25 Burns Night
31 Shooting season ends

February

14 Valentine's Day
    Shrove Tuesday

The Answers

1. b) Farmers' markets are for townies to buy food from farmers. But in fact, they were established in the wake of the foot-and-mouth disaster at the turn of the century. Villagers rallied round to try and help their local farmers by buying directly from them. Thanks to the spending power of the Notting Hill-billy who wants to prove his or her organic/local credentials, many farms have been at least propped up, if not entirely rescued, by these ventures.

2. b) Badminton is the name of the Stately Home that hosts the prestigious horse trials. But the shopping is what it's really about. All those people stuck in the hinterlands understandably get quite excited when presented with vast consumer choices after the village shop. If you hear braying – that's the shoppers, not the horses.

3. a) You may startle a family quietly having tea in their own home, despite the fact that you bought a ticket at the front door. Many a crumbling pile was rescued by the National Trust in a deal whereby

the NT covers the costs of restoration, and can earn monies from tickets, etc. but the family can still live there. This means that large numbers of aristocratic families more or less live in one room – more council estate than great estate.

4. b) and c) for this one. The best country house car boot sales, again a fairly recent idea for fundraising, has Lady Toffington clearing out her attic and sometimes even her drawing-room. However, given that many great estates have been reduced to doing this via Christie's monthly auction in order to raise dosh for the school fees, you're more likely to get the celeb cast-offs for a big charity function.

5. b) Just a very slight nod will do to greet your fellow countrymen when out on the road. And this miniscule wave is applied to everybody – to your mother as well as to the girl who served you in the post office that morning.

6. a) I just don't believe it's a country antique shop unless there's a bell tinkling. On the whole, real dealers won't rip you off, as long as you don't try to bag yourself a Canaletto for a few quid. They've had enough Americans through the door trying to buy up history in one go, and won't concern themselves with you getting over excited about a 'bargain'.

7. b) Muddy rock festivals such as Glastonbury may take place in the country, but they're what the

townies do. No self-respecting countryman would be seen headbanging at anything other than a proper festival, i.e. one held to raise money for the Countryside Alliance, with tables and tablecloths and the ever present Bryan Ferry to entertain them.

8.   A tricky one this, but I'd plump for c). The very old-fashioned would insist that you never take a present to a host, but it goes against my grain to say that anything well intentioned is 'wrong'. However, hardly anyone in the country wants to be given cut flowers, partly because they have plenty of the stuff growing outside without bringing it in, and partly because no hostess wants to faff about with vases and cellophane just as she's about to serve mini-soufflés. Make sure the chocolates are really good and expensive, though – none of your 'finest Belgian' malarkey.